NEW DEVELOPMENTS IN MEDICAL RESEARCH

CHRONIC DISEASES

THE ESCALATING DILEMMA IN DEVELOPING COUNTRIES

New Developments in Medical Research

NEW DEVELOPMENTS IN MEDICAL RESEARCH

CHRONIC DISEASES

THE ESCALATING DILEMMA IN DEVELOPING COUNTRIES

ADELIA BOVELL-BENJAMIN, PHD, CFS

NOVA BIOMEDICAL

New York

Library of Congress Cataloging-in-Publication Data

ISBN: 978-1-63321-915-1
Library of Congress Control Number: 2015955208

Published by Nova Science Publishers, Inc. † New York

Contents

List of Tables		**vii**
List of Figures		**ix**
List of Abbreviations		**xi**
Summary		**xv**
Part I: Indication		**1**
Chapter 1	Introduction	**3**
Chapter 2	Epidemiology of Chronic Diseases	**17**
Part II: Healthcare System, Governments and Non-Healthcare Systems		**39**
Chapter 3	Can Healthcare Systems in Developing Countries Cope with Chronic Diseases?	**41**
Chapter 4	Governments and Chronic Disease	**55**
Chapter 5	Non-Health Systems – Interactions and Partnerships for Chronic Disease Prevention	**65**
Part III: Chronic Disease Risk Prevention – Manipulating Common Modifiable Risk Factors		**71**
Chapter 6	Diet, Nutrition, Physical Activity and Chronic Diseases	**73**
Chapter 7	Chronic Diseases and Climate Change	**103**
Part IV: Summing up		**115**
Chapter 8	Case Studies; Evidence-Based Interventions	**117**
Chapter 9	Taking Action	**125**
Conclusion		**129**
References		**131**
Appendix A		**153**

Appendix B **167**

Appendix C **171**

Index **177**

List of Tables

Table 1. World Bank list of developing countries **11**
Table 2. Number of people with diabetes, undiagnosed diabetes and projected increase in the IDF region, 2003 **18**
Table 3. Estimated percent of chronic disease deaths in selected developing countries, 2012 **20**
Table 4. Urban population size and growth by world region **21**
Table 5. Risk factors for chronic disease **25**
Table 6. Economic burden of chronic diseases, 2011-2025 **30**
Table 7. Global economic burden of chronic diseases, 2011-2030 based on the EPIC model **32**
Table 8. Cost of type 2 diabetes in selected developing countries **36**
Table 9. Examples of the cost of kidney disease in some developed and developing countries **37**
Table 10. Comparing conventional healthcare with people-centered primary care **43**
Table 11. Attributes of effective care for chronic conditions **44**
Table 12. Percentage availability of basic diagnostic tests in primary care facilities in defined areas in eight countries, 2009/2011 **45**
Table 13. Global cardiovascular deaths attributed to sodium consumption >2 g/day in 2010, by sex, age, county income and world region **76**
Table 14. Types of salt reduction initiatives adopted by countries and regions **78**
Table 15. National efforts to reduce population salt consumption are underway in many countries **81**
Table 16. List and definition of sugar-sweetened beverages **83**
Table 17. NOURISHING framework **84-87**
Table 18. Boston Public Health Commission's point-of-purchase traffic light classification system for beverages **89**
Table 19. Under Smart Choices, foods and drinks have been classified into three categories according to their nutrition value: Green, amber and red **91**
Table 20. European and American recommended targets for cholesterol levels **97**
Table 21. Summary of life's simple seven goals from AHA **97**
Table 22. Categories of climate-change risks to health, according to causal pathway **107**

Table 23. International Diabetes Federation summary estimates for Cameroon and Jamaica, 2014 **119**
Table 24. Sample action plans for prevention/control of diabetes and hypertension in different healthcare settings 127

List of Figures

Figure 1.	Structure of the book	**4**
Figure 2.	Types of cancer	**7**
Figure 3.	Origin of cancer	**8**
Figure 4.	Benign versus malignant tumors	**8**
Figure 5.	Example of primary cancer and where they can metastasize	**9**
Figure 6.	Glucose and insulin work throughout the body	**10**
Figure 7.	Global mortality from chronic diseases	**18**
Figure 8.	Chronic diseases account for a growing share of total deaths, especially in developing regions	**19**
Figure 9.	The world population is growing and getting older	**22**
Figure 10.	World population growth in developed and developing world	**23**
Figure 11.	Poverty-chronic disease relationship	**26**
Figure 12.	The stages of nutrition transition	**27**
Figure 13.	Conceptual framework of the economic burden of diabetes	**31**
Figure 14.	Lost economic output for common chronic health problems	**34**
Figure 15.	Average annual days lost by workers with chronic condition	**34**
Figure 16.	Some major elements of direct cost-of-illness (COI)	**35**
Figure 17.	What is a health system?	**42**
Figure 18.	The chronic care model	**51**
Figure 19.	Innovate care for chronic disease framework	**52**
Figure 20.	The Expanded Chronic Care model	**53**
Figure 21.	Strategies to improve use of preventive therapies for cardiovascular health	**53**
Figure 22.	Causal web for risk factors and disease events implemented in the chronic disease prevention	**74**
Figure 23.	Mean (95% uncertainty level) sodium intakes (g/day) in 2010 in 21 global burden of diseases regions	**77**
Figure 24.	A triglyceride	**93**
Figure 25.	Comparison of the structure of four fatty acids	**94**
Figure 26.	EPA, an omega-3 fatty acid	**94**
Figure 27.	Cholesterol	**95**
Figure 28.	How the Green Prescription (GRx) works for the health profession and patient	**101**
Figure 29.	Climate change and human health	**104**

Figure 30. Conceptual framework showing three primary pathways by which climate change affect health **105**
Figure 31. Global CO_2 and greenhouse-gas emissions **105**
Figure 32. Population affected by climate-related disasters **106**
Figure 33. Cancer worldwide **108**
Figure 34. Mapping the interconnections: Type 2 diabetes and climate change **112**
Figure 35. Map of Cameroon **118**
Figure 36. Cardiovascular diseases represented in the Cardiac Center of St. Elizabeth Catholic General Hospital **120**
Figure 37. Interventions/strategies to improve healthcare for chronic diseases **130**

List of Abbreviations

AHA	American Heart Association
AIDS	Acquired immunodeficiency syndrome
Arrh	Arrhythmia
ASBs	Artificially-sweetened beverages
BCS	Building community support for diabetes care
BMI	Body mass index
bn.	Billion
CARICOM	Caribbean community
CBOs	Community-based Organizations
CCM	Chronic care model
CDC	Centers for Disease Control
CDP	Chronic disease prevention
CGI	Clinton Global Initiative
CHD	Coronary heart disease or Congestive heart failure
CHF	Congestive heart failure
CHIPs	Community Health Intervention Program
CKD	Chronic kidney disease
COI	Cost of illness
COPD	Chronic obstructive pulmonary disease
CRD	Chronic respiratory disease
CVD	Cardiovascular disease
CVS	Cerebrovascular disease
DALYs	Disability adjusted life years
DASH	Dietary approaches to stop hypertension
DNA	Deoxyribonucleic acid
ECCM	Expanded chronic care model
EPA	Eicosapentaenoic acid
EPIC	European prospective investigation into cancer and nutrition
ESKD	End stage kidney disease
FBOs	Faith-based organizations
FCTC	Framework Convention on Tobacco Control
FoPL	Front of package labeling
GDP	Gross domestic product

GDM	Gestational diabetes
GHE	Greenhouse effect
GHG	Greenhouse gas
GNI	Gross national income
HBEO	Healthy Beverage Executive Order
HD	Heart disease
HDL	High density lipoprotein
HLM	High level meeting
HTN	Hypertension
ICCC	Innovative care for chronic conditions
IDF	International Diabetes Foundation
IHD	Ischemic heart disease
KNSSP	National Health Strategic Plan
LDL	Low density lipoprotein
LMIC	Lower middle-income countries
MESA	Multi-ethnic Study of Atherosclerosis
Misc.	Miscellaneous
MTPII	National Medium Term Plan
MUFAS	Monounsaturated fatty acids
NCD	Non-communicable disease
NCI	National Cancer Institute
NGOs	Non-governmental organizations
NHANES	National Health and Nutrition Examination Survey
NHI	National Health Insurance
NIH	National Institutes of Health
ODA	Official Development Assistance
OECD	Organization for Economic Co-operation and Development
PA	Physical activity
PAAE	Physical activity energy expenditure
PAD	Peripheral arterial disease
PAHO	Pan American Health Organization
PAHs	Polycyclic aromatic hydrocarbons
PAL	Physical activity level
PHC	Primary healthcare
PUFAs	Polyunsaturated fatty acids
QoL	Quality of life
SEM	Social Ecology Model
SDG	Sustainable Development Goals
SSBs	Sugar-sweetened beverages
STEPS	Strategies for Trials Enrolment and Participation Study
T1D	Type 1 diabetes
T2D	Type 2 diabetes
TG	Triglyceride
TRIPS	The Agreement on Trade-Related Aspects of Intellectual Property Rights
UHC	Universal healthcare

UN	United Nations
UNDAF	United Nations Development Assisted Framework
UN-HABITAT	United Nations Human Settlement Program
UNIATF	United Nations Interagency Task Force on the prevention and control of non-communicable diseases
U.S.	United States
UV	Ultraviolet
UVA	Ultraviolet A
UVB	Ultraviolet B
UVC	Ultraviolet C
VBZD	Vector-borne and zoonotic diseases
WHO	World Health Organization
WTO	World Trade Organization

Summary

The central objective of the book is to provide valuable knowledge regarding the state of chronic diseases in developing countries in one place. Specifically, the book summarizes the existing literature regarding chronic diseases in developing countries; and fills significant gaps in the current state of knowledge and highlights the challenges regarding chronic diseases in developing countries.

The chronic disease epidemic is not exclusive to the developed countries; developing countries are disproportionally affected by chronic diseases. More than 80% of CVD deaths take place in developing countries, and occur almost equally in men and women (WHO, 2011a). Furthermore, the WHO reported that almost 80% of the 29 million deaths from chronic diseases occur in developing countries, with most of them occurring before the age of 60. The World Bank has also indicated that chronic diseases increasingly threaten the health and economic security of developing countries.

Over the next decade, Africa will experience the largest increases in death rates from CVD, cancer, diabetes and respiratory diseases (WHO, 2005). It is predicted that by 2030 in South Asia and Sub Saharan Africa, 21 and 18% of total deaths, respectively, would be attributed to chronic diseases. As compared to the developed countries, increases in deaths from chronic diseases are quite high in the developing countries. East Asia/Pacific, Latin America/Caribbean and Middle East/North Africa will have equally higher increases in chronic diseases death than the developed countries. The following examples demonstrate the seriousness of chronic diseases in the developing world. The information is taken from the World Health Organization's non-communicable disease (NCD) country profiles, 2014. For example, in Trinidad and Tobago, chronic diseases have been estimated to account for 80% of total deaths in 2012. In Morocco and the Bahamas, chronic diseases have been estimated to account for 75 and 72%, respectively, of all deaths.

The major determinants of chronic diseases are urbanization, aging population and globalization, these are all happening at a rate in the developing world. The major risk factors for chronic diseases are unhealthy diet, physical inactivity, and tobacco use, which are all modifiable. Individuals are more susceptible to these risk factors in situations where there is growing urbanization and globalization as experienced in many developing countries. The unparalleled rise in chronic diseases globally has been associated with the phenomenon of nutrition transition, which again is linked to high urbanization rates, and aging population among other things.

The rising prevalence of chronic diseases continues to threaten the economies of developing countries. The economic burden of chronic diseases might actually be much worse in developing countries than developed countries, but the data are still scarce. Projections reveal that more than $7 trillion will be lost from the four major chronic diseases in low-middle-income countries (LMIC) between 2011 to 2025; averaging roughly US$500 billion (bn.) annually. The presence and growing prevalence of chronic diseases in developing countries will continue to present primary stumbling blocks to economic growth. Global estimates for CVD in 2010 were US$863 bn., which is projected to increase to US$1,044 bn. in 2030. The number is equally daunting for diabetes; the global cost was approximately US$500 bn. in 2010. Intangible cost such as pain, anxiety, inconvenience and other factors which diminish QoL are equally enormous as direct and indirect cost, and are frequently unquantifiable. In Burkina Faso, financial difficulties increased by 50% in households affected by chronic disease. The economic burden of chronic disease emphasizes the need for initiatives to prevent and control chronic disease prevalence and their devastating complications.

Various models for chronic disease management have been propositioned and executed globally. Research has indicated that the implementation of the CCM in developed countries verified significant correlations between certain elements of the CCM and better health outcomes. The ICCC gives greater emphasis to community and policy aspects of improving health care for chronic disease. The ECCM extends the role of healthcare systems and providers outside clinical settings. Developing countries must begin to select the model(s) most appropriate to their situation and begin to implement aspects of these models if they are to curb the rising chronic disease problem, which is threatening their sustainable development.

Governments must take the lead in the fight against chronic diseases, building the case for intervention; encouraging advocacy and developing social marketing campaigns; and making interventions to reduce poor dietary intake and protect consumer health. The literature provides a vast majority of suggested interventions, which governments, if they have the political will could adopt to meet their countries' needs.

WHO has global recommendations on physical activity for health for member countries. Only a minority of Africans engage in vigorous physical activity. The same is true for Iran. Efforts are underway in some countries, such as New Zealand, South Africa and the U.S. to increase physical activity levels. A variety of cost-effective chronic disease interventions have been documented for all regions of the world, including sub-Saharan Africa. Each country, regardless of the level of its resources, has the potential to make significant improvements in chronic disease prevention and control, and to take steps towards achieving the global goal. Indeed, resources are necessary, but a large amount can be achieved for little cost, for example altering diets and increasing physical activity.

In sum, the effects of climate change on health are likely to be predominantly negative and impact most heavily on developing countries where the capacity to adapt is weakest. For example, there is less access to effective health system infrastructure in the developing countries. It is predicted that developing countries would bear 80% of the climate change burden. The climate change/cancer linkage has been associated with exposure to toxic chemicals, and depletion of the stratospheric ozone. Increases in respiratory diseases have also been reported after flooding in developing and developed countries.

There is increasing evidence that air pollution contributes to an unacceptable burden of chronic disease and premature mortality, especially from respiratory and cardiovascular causes. Climate change may aggravate CVD by intensifying heat stress, increasing the body burden of airborne particulates, and modifying the distribution of zoonotic vectors, which trigger infectious diseases linked to CVD. For example, CVD hospital admissions increased with heat, and dysrhythmias were predominantly associated with extreme cold. Disasters such as floods and storms could further threaten the fragile health systems in developing countries, and weaken capacity for diabetes prevention and management. Mitigation policies should be put into place to reduce the effects of climate change on chronic disease in developing countries. Governments should ensure that populations better understand the relationship between climate change and chronic disease for improved prevention and management of chronic diseases.

Out-of-pocket payments for treatment are required to sustain the healthcare system in Cameroon. The catastrophic effect of out-of-pocket payments on families has been discussed throughout the book. Healthcare systems in developing countries must be improved if the halt in chronic disease is to be realized. Throughout the book, various interventions/strategies have been described, which could improve health care for chronic disease. Although some progress has been made, developing countries are still facing an escalating burden from chronic diseases, which is impacting negatively on sustainable development. Developing countries urgently need to scale up chronic disease prevention and control programs to circumvent this escalating dilemma. The role of governments in developing countries is critical to the development and implementation of well-informed risk-factor chronic disease prevention and control programs. Reallocation of healthcare budgets, policy and system changes, partnerships with NGOs and food industry are essential to reduce chronic disease risk in populations.

Populations in developing countries need to be more aware about basic prevention measures. Governments, private entities, stakeholders, health professionals, civil societies, all must support chronic disease prevention/control by legislation, building human resource capacity for healthcare workers, public education to reduce dietary fat, salt and sugar, food pricing policies, tobacco control, food formulation and changes as discussed to healthcare delivery systems. Chronic disease prevention/control needs to be placed higher on the political agenda of developing countries; policy makers should be fully informed with the up-to-date evidence about the burden and far reaching impacts of chronic diseases. Governments must support the effort with the necessary resources and firm commitment. Private entities, community members, individuals, families and family members must join in the coordinated and focused effort to halt the escalating dilemma of chronic diseases in developing countries.

Part I: Indication

Chapter 1

Introduction

Scope

This book creates awareness about the chronic disease problem in developing countries by outlining the magnitude and dilemma (that is the double burden of disease), putting it in context, while examining the burden, best practices, government policies, prevention, the direction and the way forward using an integrated approach. The book relates chronic diseases to climate change and sustainable development as have not been done before. It points out the need for involvement of the non-health sector, discusses the partnership with the food industry and other stakeholders for better understanding and solutions to the dilemma of the escalating problem of chronic diseases. It highlights published literature to advocate urgent action to prevent the problem from further escalating, and summarizes a number of strategies, policies and recommendations. Although the book discusses chronic diseases in the developing world, it tends to focus more on diabetes (one of the four main classes of chronic diseases), Africa and the Caribbean region to illustrate the escalating problem in developing countries. The book is divided into three parts. Part 1, chapter 1 describes the scope of the book, defines selected chronic diseases, and shows the classification of developing countries. The epidemiology of chronic disease, determinants, risk factors, nutrition transition and the economic burden of chronic diseases are described in Chapter 2. Part II discusses healthcare systems in developing countries. The structure of the book is shown in Figure 1.

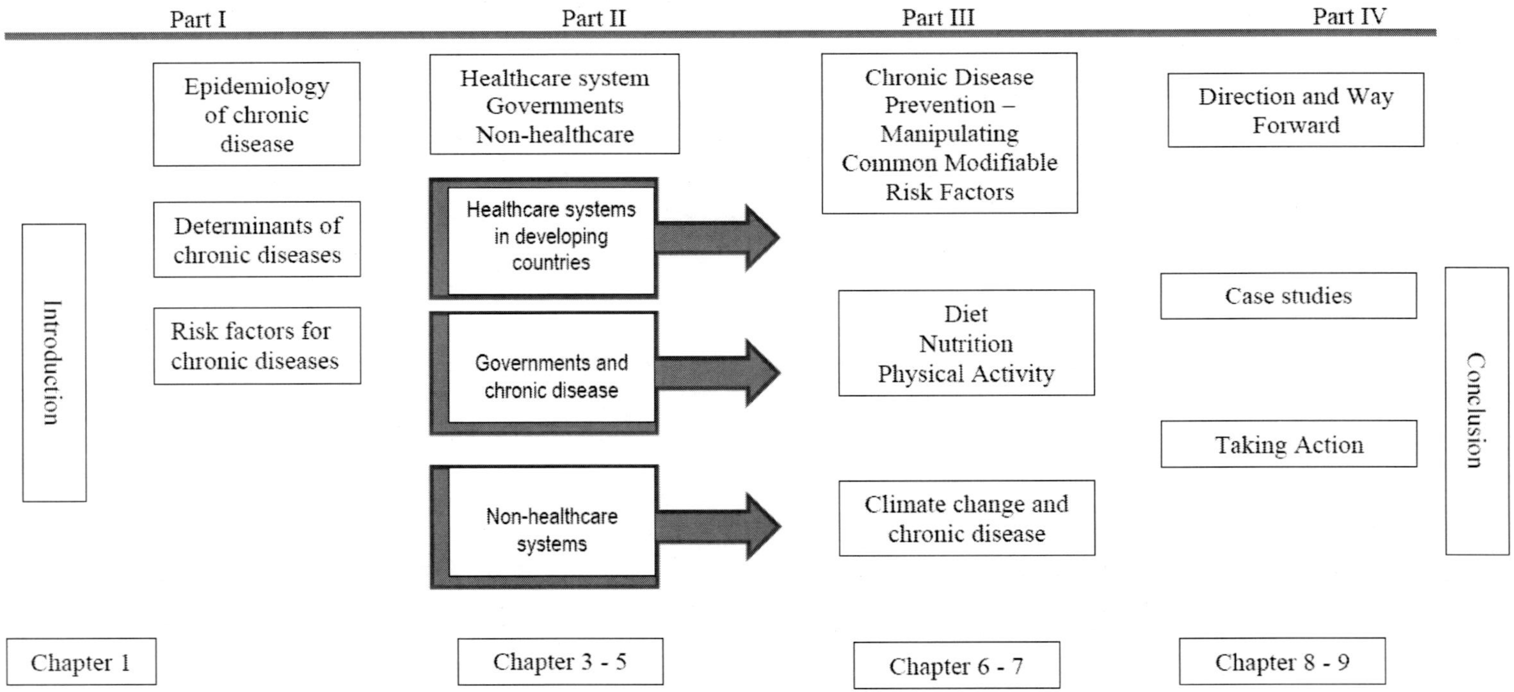

Figure 1. Structure of the Book.

The book is applicable for use by academia, health educators, health professionals who practice, study or teach chronic diseases, doctors, medical students and researchers; planners in government agencies, nutritionists, dietitians, students in the biological and social sciences, food industry, insurance companies, pharmaceutical industry, ministries of health, non-governmental organizations (NGOs), community-based organizations (CBOs), faith-based organizations (FBOs), and chronic disease organizations. Overall, the book has some advantages over competitive publications because it focuses on developing countries, where the problem is escalating; the burden of chronic diseases is higher; and there is a double burden of disease (that is, infectious and non-communicable diseases). Also, this book is much more comprehensive in topic areas and would appeal to a wider audience than others on the market.

The central objective of the book is to provide valuable knowledge regarding the state of chronic diseases in developing countries in one place. Specifically, the book summarizes the existing literature regarding chronic diseases in developing countries; and fills significant gaps in the current state of knowledge and highlights the challenges regarding chronic diseases in developing countries.

Methods

This book is based upon a comprehensive review of the literature available on chronic diseases; however, it is not all-inclusive. A wide range of medical, environmental, governmental, international and scientific databases such as PubMed and Science Direct had been searched to track the current, past and future status of chronic diseases and healthcare systems in developed and developing countries. The electronic searches were supplemented by hand searching in some instances. Various Internet engines were searched for web pages of International Organizations such as the World Health Organization and the World Bank, which have information, recommendations, policies and toolkits for chronic diseases.

A basic literature search with various combinations of keywords from the topic such as 'chronic diseases'; 'global state of chronic disease'; and 'cost of chronic disease' yielded many results. The Internet search led to project documents (reports, proposals and plans), as well as to online toolkits, reports, policy documents, materials from NGOs, scientific publications, working papers, theses and online papers from academic institutions, and databases. After having surveyed the literature, the amount of published work relevant to chronic diseases especially in developing countries is impressive and enough to jumpstart the world into action to halt the escalating predicament of chronic diseases.

Definitions

Chronic Disease

Chronic diseases are also referred to as non-communicable diseases or 'diseases of lifestyle'. Several definitions have been used in the literature for chronic diseases. According to Daar et al. (2007), chronic diseases are conditions which are known to affect individuals over an extensive period of time, and for which there are no known causative agents that are transmitted from one individual to another. WHO (2005) explains chronic diseases as a set of conditions with important shared features including: i) chronic disease epidemics take decades to become fully established, that is, they have their origins at young ages; ii) their long duration provides many opportunities for prevention; and iii) they require a long-term and systematic approach to treatment. Al-Maskari (2010) outlines chronic diseases as having shared risk factors similar to prolonged exposure to smoking, unhealthy diet and physical inactivity. Higuchi (2010) defines chronic disease as shrinking the quality of life in patients, causing premature death, and leading to other adverse consequences. In a nutshell, chronic conditions have insistent or habitual health outcomes, which last for years. They are illnesses or impediments, which cannot be cured, but can be prevented. In this book, the WHO (2005) definition of chronic diseases has been adopted.

The literature groups the most prominent chronic diseases into four main classes: cardiovascular diseases (CVD); cancer; chronic respiratory disease (CRD); and diabetes (Nugent 2008). However, there are other chronic diseases such as mental illness, vision and hearing loss, and digestive diseases such as cirrhosis (Suhrcke et al., 2006; Bloom et al., 2011). A brief description of the most common chronic diseases discussed in this book follows.

Cardiovascular Disease (CVD)

The World Health Organization describes CVD as a group of disorders of the heart and blood vessels, which encompass: i) coronary heart disease (CHD), which affects the blood vessels supplying the heart muscle; ii) cerebrovascular disease (CVS) affects the blood vessels supplying the brain; and peripheral arterial disease (PAD) affects the blood vessels supplying the arms and legs; iii) rheumatic heart disease describes damage to the heart muscle and valves from rheumatic fever, caused by streptococcal bacteria; iv) congenital heart disease is malformations of heart structure existing at birth; and v) deep vein thrombosis and pulmonary embolism are blood clots in the leg veins, which can dislodge and move to the heart and lungs. WHO further describes heart attacks and strokes as usually acute events mainly caused by a blockage that prevents blood from flowing to the heart or brain. The most common reason is a build-up of fatty deposits on the inner walls of the blood vessels. Strokes can be caused by bleeding from a blood vessel in the brain or by blood clots.

Cancer

Cancer is the Latin word for crab, which was used to mean a malignancy, possibly because of the crab-like tenaciousness malignant tumors show in grasping the tissues they invade. Cancer is also known as malignancy, a malignant tumor, or a neoplasm. Cancer describes a large group of diseases, which affects any part of the body. It is characterized by the rapid growth of abnormal cells, which can invade parts of the body and spread to other organs (Bloom et al., 2011). Most cancers are named for the organ or type of cell in which they start. For example, cancer that begins in the colon is called colon cancer; cancer that begins in melanocytes of the skin is called melanoma.

According to the National Cancer Institute of the United States (U.S.), cancer types can be grouped into broader categories. The five main categories of cancer include: i) Carcinoma (which has a number of subtypes) begins in the skin or tissues which line or cover internal organs; ii) Sarcoma begins in bone, cartilage, fat, muscle, blood vessels, or other connective or supportive tissue; iii) Leukemia starts in blood-forming tissue such as the bone marrow and causes large numbers of abnormal blood cells to be produced and enter the blood; iv) Lymphoma and myeloma are cancers that begin in the cells of the immune system; and v) Central nervous system cancers originate in the tissues of the brain and spinal cord. Figure 2 shows some of the different types of cancer.

Cancers begin in cells, the body's basic unit of life. The body is made up of many types of cells. These cells grow and divide in a controlled way to produce more cells as they are needed to keep the body healthy. Normally, old or damaged cells die and are replaced with new cells. However, sometimes this orderly process goes wrong. Deoxyribonucleic acid (DNA), the genetic material of a cell can become damaged or changed, producing mutations, which alter normal cell growth and division. This prevents cells from dying when they should, and promotes the growth of new cells when the body does not need them. The extra cells may form a mass of tissue called a tumor (Figure 3). Tumors can be benign or malignant (Figure 4). Benign tumors are not cancerous. They can often be removed, and, in most cases, do not return. Cells in benign tumors do not spread to other parts of the body. On the other hand, malignant tumors are cancerous. Cells in these tumors can invade nearby tissues and spread to other parts of the body. The spread of cancer from one part of the body to another is called metastasis (Figure 5). Some cancers do not form tumors, for example, leukemia is a cancer of the bone marrow and blood.

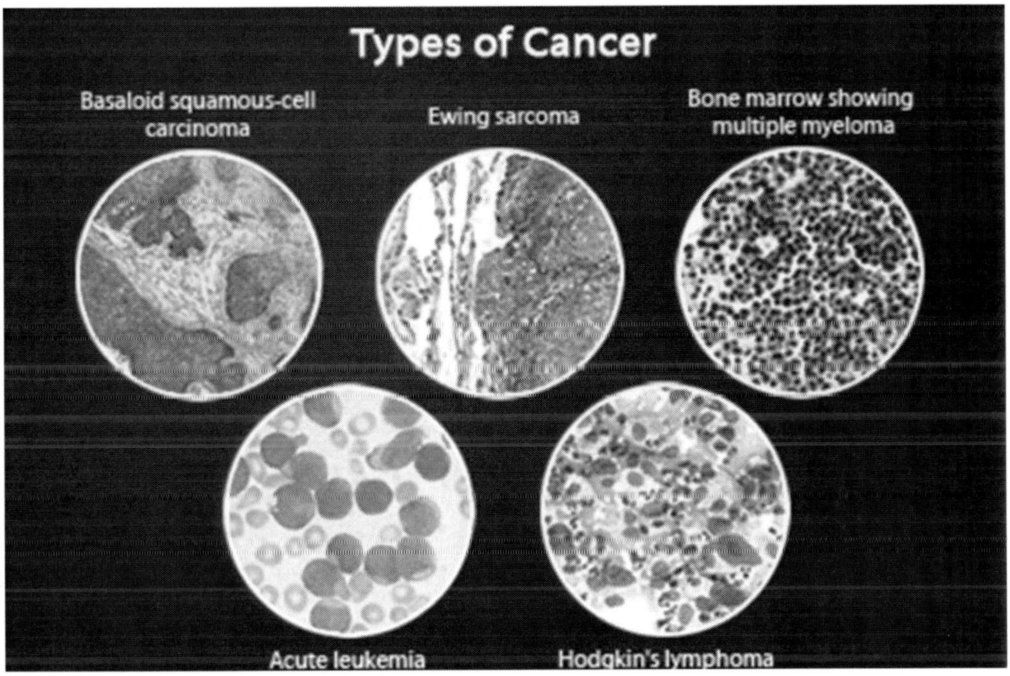

Figure 2. Types of cancer Available at: http://www.medicinenet.com.

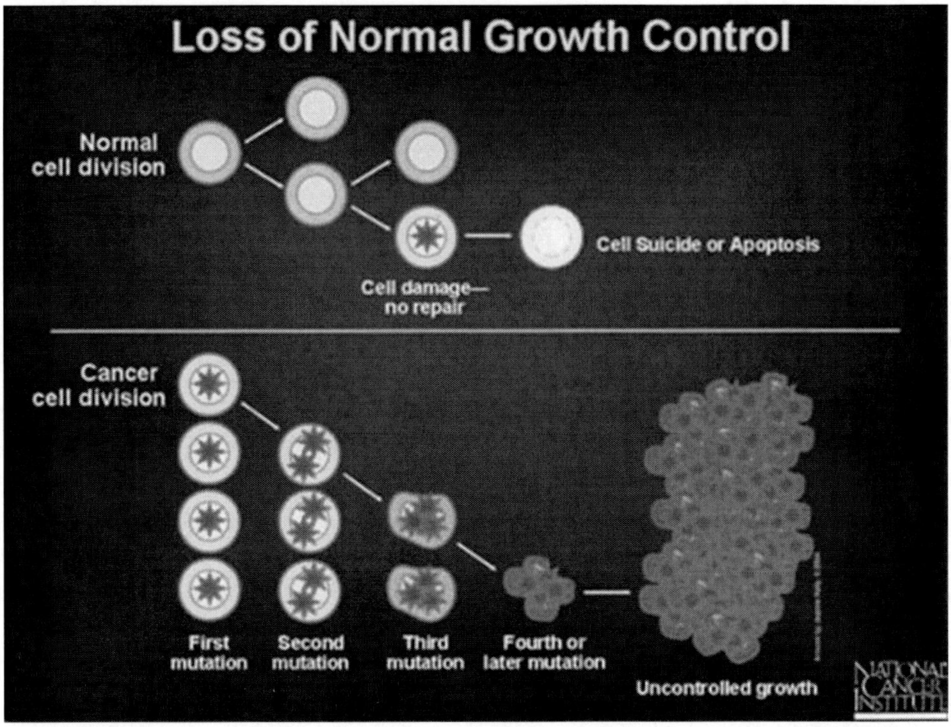

Figure 3. Origin of cancer (loss of normal growth control); available at: http://www.medicinenet.com.

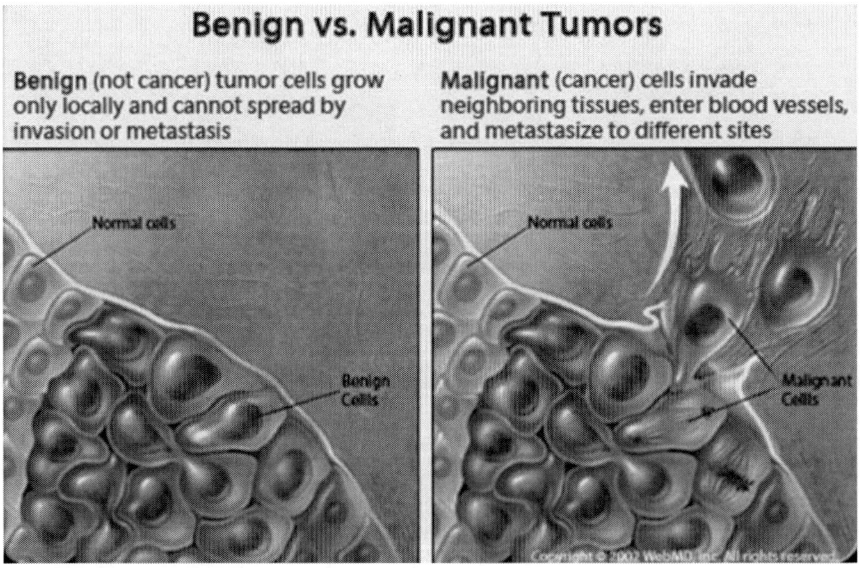

Figure 4. Benign versus malignant tumors; available at: http://www.medicinenet.com.

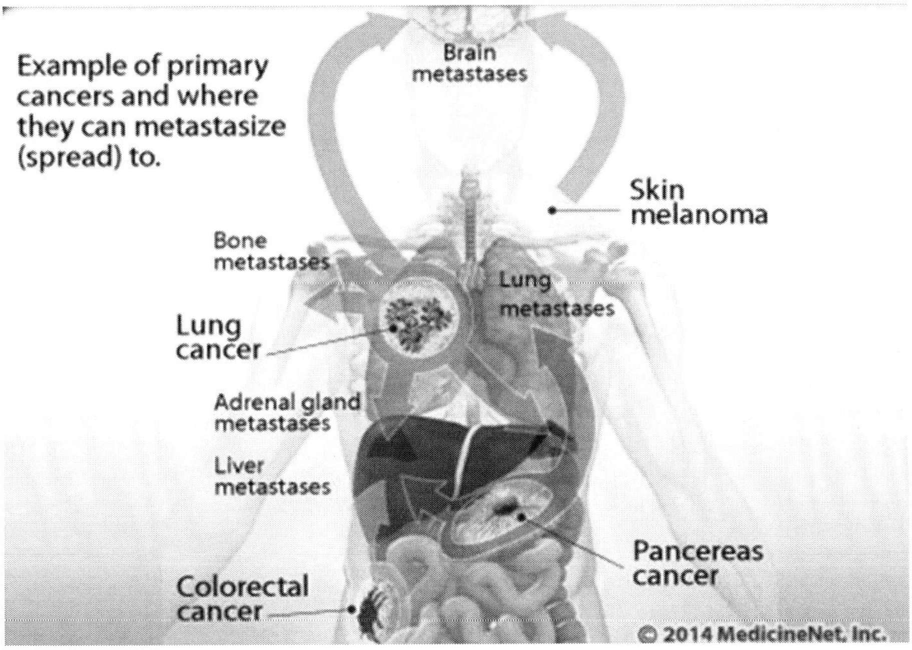

Figure 5. Example of primary cancer and where they can metastasize to.
Available at: http://www.medicinenet.com.

Chronic Respiratory Disease (CRD)

Chronic respiratory diseases affect the airways and other structures of the lung. Some common respiratory diseases are asthma, chronic obstructive pulmonary disease (COPD) and respiratory allergies (Bloom et al., 2011). Asthma is a disease characterized by recurrent attacks of breathlessness and wheezing, which vary in severity and frequency from person to person. Asthma attacks all age groups but often starts in childhood. This condition is due to inflammation of the air passages in the lungs, and affects the sensitivity of the nerve endings in the airways so they become easily irritated. In an attack, the lining of the passages swell causing the airways to narrow and reducing the flow of air in and out of the lungs. COPD includes a group of chronic lung diseases, which limits airflow in the lungs. The older terms, such as chronic bronchitis and emphysema, previously used, have now been replaced with the COPD diagnosis. The most common symptoms of COPD are breathlessness, excessive sputum production, and a chronic cough. COPD is a life threatening lung disease that may progressively lead to death.

Diabetes

The word diabetes is from the Greek word meaning a siphon because of the excessive urination associated with the condition. According to WHO, diabetes mellitus describes a metabolic disorder of multiple etiologies. Diabetes is characterized by chronic hyperglycemia with disturbances of carbohydrate, fat and protein metabolism resulting from defects in insulin secretion, insulin action, or both. The effects of diabetes mellitus include long-term damage, dysfunction and failure of various organs (WHO, 1999).

There are two main types of diabetes mellitus: i) Type 1 diabetes (T1D), which usually develops in childhood and adolescence. In T1D, individuals require lifelong insulin injections for survival; ii) Type 2 diabetes (T2D) usually develops in adulthood, and is related to obesity, physical inactivity, and unhealthy diets. T2D is the more common type of diabetes (representing 90% of diabetes cases globally). Treatment may involve lifestyle changes and weight loss alone, or oral medications or even insulin injections; and iii) Gestational diabetes (a state of hyperglycemia, which develops during pregnancy). Intermediate states of hyperglycemia (impaired fasting glucose or impaired glucose tolerance), which can progress to diabetes have also been defined in gestational diabetes. Regulation of the blood sugar levels in the body is centered on the hormone insulin, which is released from cells located in the pancreas. Insulin speeds up the transfer of sugar from the blood and delivers it to the muscles, liver and fat tissues where it is used as fuel or stored for future use by the body (Figure 6).

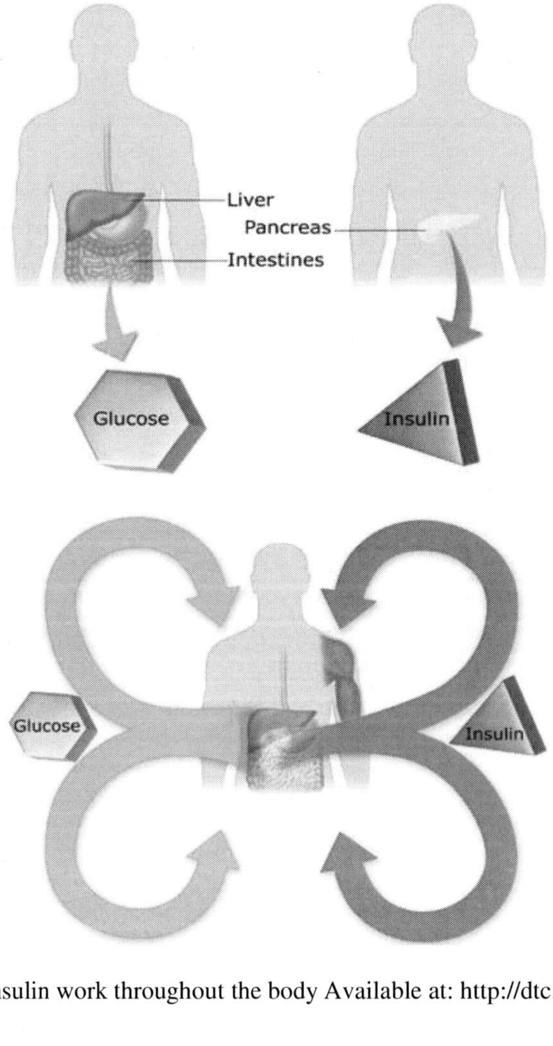

Figure 6. Glucose and insulin work throughout the body Available at: http://dtc.ucsf.edu.

Classifying Developing Countries

Developing countries or economies are defined according to their Gross National Income (GNI) per capita per year. Each year on July 1, The World Bank revises the classification of the world's economies based on estimates of GNI for the previous year. The 2015 World Bank income classifications by GNI per capita are: i) low income ≤ US$1,035; ii) lower middle income: US$1,036 to $4,085; iii) upper middle income: US$4,086 to $12,615; and iv) high income ≥ US$12,616. In this book, the term country is used interchangeably with *economy, while t*he term *developing* is used to denote low-, middle- and high-income countries. The World Bank's classification of the developing countries is shown in Table 1.

Table 1. World Bank List of Economies/Developing Countries
***Available at: https://muse.jhu.edu/about/order/wdi2015.pdf* (accessed 8/27/15)**

Economy	Region	Income Group
Afghanistan	South Asia	Low income
Albania	Europe & Central Asia	Upper middle income
Algeria	Middle East & North Africa	Upper middle income
American Samoa	East Asia & Pacific	Upper middle income
Andorra	Europe & Central Asia	High income: nonOECD
Angola	Sub-Saharan Africa	Upper middle income
Antigua and Barbuda	Latin America & Caribbean	High income: nonOECD
Argentina	Latin America & Caribbean	**High income: nonOECD**
Armenia	Europe & Central Asia	Lower middle income
Aruba	Latin America & Caribbean	High income: nonOECD
Australia	East Asia & Pacific	High income: OECD
Austria	Europe & Central Asia	High income: OECD
Azerbaijan	Europe & Central Asia	Upper middle income
Bahamas, The	Latin America & Caribbean	High income: nonOECD
Bahrain	Middle East & North Africa	High income: nonOECD
Bangladesh	South Asia	**Lower middle income**
Barbados	Latin America & Caribbean	High income: nonOECD
Belarus	Europe & Central Asia	Upper middle income
Belgium	Europe & Central Asia	High income: OECD
Belize	Latin America & Caribbean	Upper middle income
Benin	Sub-Saharan Africa	Low income
Bermuda	North America	High income: nonOECD
Bhutan	South Asia	Lower middle income
Bolivia	Latin America & Caribbean	Lower middle income
Bosnia and Herzegovina	Europe & Central Asia	Upper middle income
Botswana	Sub-Saharan Africa	Upper middle income
Brazil	Latin America & Caribbean	Upper middle income
Brunei Darussalam	East Asia & Pacific	High income: nonOECD
Bulgaria	Europe & Central Asia	Upper middle income
Burkina Faso	Sub-Saharan Africa	Low income
Burundi	Sub-Saharan Africa	Low income
Cabo Verde	Sub-Saharan Africa	Lower middle income
Cambodia	East Asia & Pacific	Low income
Cameroon	Sub-Saharan Africa	Lower middle income
Canada	North America	High income: OECD

Table 1. (Continued)

Economy	Region	Income Group
Cayman Islands	Latin America & Caribbean	High income: nonOECD
Central African Republic	Sub-Saharan Africa	Low income
Chad	Sub-Saharan Africa	Low income
Channel Islands	Europe & Central Asia	High income: nonOECD
Chile	Latin America & Caribbean	High income: OECD
China	East Asia & Pacific	Upper middle income
Colombia	Latin America & Caribbean	Upper middle income
Comoros	Sub-Saharan Africa	Low income
Congo, Dem. Rep.	Sub-Saharan Africa	Low income
Congo, Rep.	Sub-Saharan Africa	Lower middle income
Costa Rica	Latin America & Caribbean	Upper middle income
Côte d'Ivoire	Sub-Saharan Africa	Lower middle income
Croatia	Europe & Central Asia	High income: nonOECD
Cuba	Latin America & Caribbean	Upper middle income
Curaçao	Latin America & Caribbean	High income: nonOECD
Croatia	Europe & Central Asia	High income: nonOECD
Cuba	Latin America & Caribbean	Upper middle income
Curaçao	Latin America & Caribbean	High income: nonOECD
Cyprus	Europe & Central Asia	High income: nonOECD
Czech Republic	Europe & Central Asia	High income: OECD
Denmark	Europe & Central Asia	High income: OECD
Djibouti	Middle East & North Africa	Lower middle income
Dominica	Latin America & Caribbean	Upper middle income
Dominican Republic	Latin America & Caribbean	Upper middle income
Ecuador	Latin America & Caribbean	Upper middle income
Egypt, Arab Rep.	Middle East & North Africa	Lower middle income
El Salvador	Latin America & Caribbean	Lower middle income
Equatorial Guinea	Sub-Saharan Africa	High income: nonOECD
Eritrea	Sub-Saharan Africa	Low income
Estonia	Europe & Central Asia	High income: OECD
Ethiopia	Sub-Saharan Africa	Low income
Faeroe Islands	Europe & Central Asia	High income: nonOECD
Fiji	East Asia & Pacific	Upper middle income
Finland	Europe & Central Asia	High income: OECD
France	Europe & Central Asia	High income: OECD
French Polynesia	East Asia & Pacific	High income: nonOECD
Gabon	Sub-Saharan Africa	Upper middle income
Gambia, The	Sub-Saharan Africa	Low income
Georgia	Europe & Central Asia	Lower middle income
Germany	Europe & Central Asia	High income: OECD
Ghana	Sub-Saharan Africa	Lower middle income
Greece	Europe & Central Asia	High income: OECD
Greenland	Europe & Central Asia	High income: nonOECD
Grenada	Latin America & Caribbean	Upper middle income
Guam	East Asia & Pacific	High income: nonOECD
Guatemala	Latin America & Caribbean	Lower middle income
Guinea	Sub-Saharan Africa	Low income
Guinea-Bissau	Sub-Saharan Africa	Low income
Guyana	Latin America & Caribbean	Lower middle income

Economy	Region	Income Group
Haiti	Latin America & Caribbean	Low income
Honduras	Latin America & Caribbean	Lower middle income
Hong Kong SAR, China	East Asia & Pacific	High income: nonOECD
Hungary	Europe & Central Asia	**High income: OECD**
Iceland	Europe & Central Asia	High income: OECD
India	South Asia	Lower middle income
Indonesia	East Asia & Pacific	Lower middle income
Iran, Islamic Rep.	Middle East & North Africa	Upper middle income
Iraq	Middle East & North Africa	Upper middle income
Ireland	Europe & Central Asia	High income: OECD
Isle of Man	Europe & Central Asia	High income: nonOECD
Israel	Middle East & North Africa	High income: OECD
Italy	Europe & Central Asia	High income: OECD
Jamaica	Latin America & Caribbean	Upper middle income
Japan	East Asia & Pacific	High income: OECD
Jordan	Middle East & North Africa	Upper middle income
Kazakhstan	Europe & Central Asia	Upper middle income
Kenya	Sub-Saharan Africa	**Lower middle income**
Kiribati	East Asia & Pacific	Lower middle income
Korea, Dem. Rep.	East Asia & Pacific	Low income
Korea, Rep.	East Asia & Pacific	High income: OECD
Kosovo	Europe & Central Asia	Lower middle income
Kuwait	Middle East & North Africa	High income: nonOECD
Kyrgyz Republic	Europe & Central Asia	Lower middle income
Lao PDR	East Asia & Pacific	Lower middle income
Latvia	Europe & Central Asia	High income: nonOECD
Lebanon	Middle East & North Africa	Upper middle income
Lesotho	Sub-Saharan Africa	Lower middle income
Liberia	Sub-Saharan Africa	Low income
Libya	Middle East & North Africa	Upper middle income
Liechtenstein	Europe & Central Asia	High income: nonOECD
Lithuania	Europe & Central Asia	High income: nonOECD
Luxembourg	Europe & Central Asia	High income: OECD
Macao SAR, China	East Asia & Pacific	High income: nonOECD
Macedonia, FYR	Europe & Central Asia	Upper middle income
Madagascar	Sub-Saharan Africa	Low income
Malawi	Sub-Saharan Africa	Low income
Malaysia	East Asia & Pacific	Upper middle income
Maldives	South Asia	Upper middle income
Mali	Sub-Saharan Africa	Low income
Malta	Middle East & North Africa	High income: nonOECD
Marshall Islands	East Asia & Pacific	Upper middle income
Mauritania	Sub-Saharan Africa	Lower middle income
Mauritius	Sub-Saharan Africa	Upper middle income
Mexico	Latin America & Caribbean	Upper middle income
Micronesia, Fed. Sts.	East Asia & Pacific	Lower middle income
Moldova	Europe & Central Asia	Lower middle income
Monaco	Europe & Central Asia	High income: nonOECD
Mongolia	East Asia & Pacific	**Upper middle income**
Montenegro	Europe & Central Asia	Upper middle income
Morocco	Middle East & North Africa	Lower middle income

Table 1. (Continued)

Economy	Region	Income Group
Mozambique	Sub-Saharan Africa	Low income
Myanmar	East Asia & Pacific	**Lower middle income**
Namibia	Sub-Saharan Africa	Upper middle income
Nepal	South Asia	Low income
Netherlands	Europe & Central Asia	High income: OECD
New Caledonia	East Asia & Pacific	High income: nonOECD
New Zealand	East Asia & Pacific	High income: OECD
Nicaragua	Latin America & Caribbean	Lower middle income
Niger	Sub-Saharan Africa	Low income
Nigeria	Sub-Saharan Africa	Lower middle income
Northern Mariana Islands	East Asia & Pacific	High income: nonOECD
Norway	Europe & Central Asia	High income: OECD
Oman	Middle East & North Africa	High income: nonOECD
Pakistan	South Asia	Lower middle income
Palau	East Asia & Pacific	Upper middle income
Panama	Latin America & Caribbean	Upper middle income
Papua New Guinea	East Asia & Pacific	Lower middle income
Paraguay	Latin America & Caribbean	**Upper middle income**
Peru	Latin America & Caribbean	Upper middle income
Philippines	East Asia & Pacific	Lower middle income
Poland	Europe & Central Asia	High income: OECD
Portugal	Europe & Central Asia	High income: OECD
Puerto Rico	Latin America & Caribbean	High income: nonOECD
Qatar	Middle East & North Africa	High income: nonOECD
Romania	Europe & Central Asia	Upper middle income
Russian Federation	Europe & Central Asia	High income: nonOECD
Rwanda	Sub-Saharan Africa	Low income
Samoa	East Asia & Pacific	Lower middle income
San Marino	Europe & Central Asia	High income: nonOECD
São Tomé and Principe	Sub-Saharan Africa	Lower middle income
Saudi Arabia	Middle East & North Africa	High income: nonOECD
Senegal	Sub-Saharan Africa	Lower middle income
Serbia	Europe & Central Asia	Upper middle income
Seychelles	Sub-Saharan Africa	**High income: nonOECD**
Sierra Leone	Sub-Saharan Africa	Low income
Singapore	East Asia & Pacific	High income: nonOECD
Saint Maarten (Dutch part)	Latin America & Caribbean	High income: nonOECD
Slovak Republic	Europe & Central Asia	High income: OECD
Slovenia	Europe & Central Asia	High income: OECD
Solomon Islands	East Asia & Pacific	Lower middle income
Somalia	Sub-Saharan Africa	Low income
South Africa	Sub-Saharan Africa	Upper middle income
South Sudan	Sub-Saharan Africa	Low income
Spain	Europe & Central Asia	High income: OECD
Sri Lanka	South Asia	Lower middle income
St. Kitts and Nevis	Latin America & Caribbean	High income: nonOECD
St. Lucia	Latin America & Caribbean	Upper middle income
St. Martin (French part)	Latin America & Caribbean	High income: nonOECD

Economy	Region	Income Group
St. Vincent and the Grenadines	Latin America & Caribbean	Upper middle income
Sudan	Sub-Saharan Africa	Lower middle income
Suriname	Latin America & Caribbean	Upper middle income
Swaziland	Sub-Saharan Africa	Lower middle income
Sweden	Europe & Central Asia	High income: OECD
Switzerland	Europe & Central Asia	High income: OECD
Syrian Arab Republic	Middle East & North Africa	Lower middle income
Taiwan, China	East Asia & Pacific	High income: nonOECD
Tajikistan	Europe & Central Asia	**Lower middle income**
Tanzania	Sub-Saharan Africa	Low income
Thailand	East Asia & Pacific	Upper middle income
Timor-Leste	East Asia & Pacific	Lower middle income
Togo	Sub-Saharan Africa	Low income
Tonga	East Asia & Pacific	Upper middle income
Trinidad and Tobago	Latin America & Caribbean	High income: nonOECD
Tunisia	Middle East & North Africa	Upper middle income
Turkey	Europe & Central Asia	Upper middle income
Turkmenistan	Europe & Central Asia	Upper middle income
Turks and Caicos Islands	Latin America & Caribbean	High income: nonOECD
Tuvalu	East Asia & Pacific	Upper middle income
Uganda	Sub-Saharan Africa	Low income
Ukraine	Europe & Central Asia	Lower middle income
United Arab Emirates	Middle East & North Africa	High income: nonOECD
United Kingdom	Europe & Central Asia	High income: OECD
United States	North America	High income: OECD
Uruguay	Latin America & Caribbean	High income: nonOECD
Uzbekistan	Europe & Central Asia	Lower middle income
Vanuatu	East Asia & Pacific	Lower middle income
Venezuela, RB	Latin America & Caribbean	High income: nonOECD
Vietnam	East Asia & Pacific	Lower middle income
Virgin Islands (U.S.)	Latin America & Caribbean	High income: nonOECD
West Bank and Gaza	Middle East & North Africa	Lower middle income
Yemen, Rep.	Middle East & North Africa	Lower middle income
Zambia	Sub-Saharan Africa	Lower middle income
Zimbabwe	Sub-Saharan Africa	Low income

This table classifies all World Bank member economies, and all other economies with populations of more than 30,000. For operational and analytical purposes, economies are divided among income groups according to 2014 gross national income (GNI) per capita, calculated using the World Bank Atlas method. The groups are: low income, $1,045 or less; lower middle income, $1,046–4,125; upper middle income, $4,126–12,735; and high income, $12,736 or more. Other analytical groups based on geographic regions are also used. Geographic classifications in this table cover all income levels; data reported for geographic regions may cover low- and middle-income economies only. Low-income and middle-income economies are sometimes referred to as developing economies. The use of the term is convenient; it is not intended to imply that all economies in the group are experiencing similar development or that other economies have reached a preferred or final stage of development. Classification by income does not necessarily reflect development status. Lending category: IDA countries are those that had a per capita income in 2014 of less than $1,215 and lack the financial ability to borrow from IBRD. IDA loans are deeply concessional—interest-free loans and grants for programs aimed at boosting economic growth and improving living conditions. IBRD loans are noncessional. Blend countries are eligible for IDA loans because of their low per capita incomes but are also eligible for IBRD loans because they are financially creditworthy. Note: Income classifications set on 1 July 2015 remain in effect until 1 July 2016. Lithuania joined the euro area on 1 January 2015.

Table 1 classifies all World Bank member economies and all other economies with populations of more than 30,000. Economies are divided among income groups according to 2014 gross national income (GNI) per capita, calculated using the World Bank Atlas method. The groups are: low income, $1,045 or less; lower middle income, $1,046–4,125; upper middle income, $4,126–12,735; and high income, $12,736 or more. Geographic classifications in the table cover all income levels; data reported for geographic regions may cover low- and middle-income economies only.

In reviewing the definitions of the four main classes of chronic diseases (CVD, cancer, CRD, and diabetes), it is clear that they usually share the same underlying root cause, for example, low physical activity levels and inadequate diets. Evidence-based, effective approaches used to prevent and control these conditions could be adopted and interchanged among them. It should be emphasized that there are other types of chronic diseases such as mental illness. Low-income and middle-income economies or countries are sometimes referred to as developing economies or countries. The World Bank stresses that classification by income does not necessarily reflect development status, and this should be borne in mind by the reader.

Chapter 2

Epidemiology of Chronic Diseases

Background

The World Health Organization (WHO) predicted deaths from chronic diseases to rise by 15% between 2010 and 2020, with jumps of over 20% in Africa and South-East Asia. For example, the number of people in the developing world with diabetes will increase by more than 2.5-fold, from 84 million in 1995 to 228 million in 2025. Furthermore, the WHO reported that almost 80% of deaths from chronic diseases now occur in developing countries, where most of the world's population resides. Chronic diseases negatively affect the quality of life (QoL) of affected individuals; contribute to premature death; create huge economic burdens on families, communities, and societies in general. Unless urgent action is taken, 41 and 55 million people will die of a chronic disease in 2015 and 2030, respectively (WHO, 2013).

Globally, chronic diseases are a great and growing health problem and the largest cause of deaths (Figure 7). By 2020, the WHO predicts that chronic diseases will be responsible for 73% of all deaths, and 60% of the global burden of disease, with escalations of over 20% in Africa and South-East Asia. For example, in 2008, an estimated 17.3 million people died from CVDs, which were roughly 30% of all global deaths (WHO, 2011a). Cancer accounted for 8.2 million deaths in 2012 (Globocan 2012). The developing world accounts for 70% of the world's cancer deaths (Globocan, 2012). It is predicted that annual cancer deaths will increase to 22 million over the next 20 years (Globocan 2012).

The International Diabetes Federation (IDF) indicates that 382 million people have diabetes, and there is a projected increase to more than 592 million in 2035 (Aguiree et al., 2013). Of the total number affected by diabetes, more than 80% of diabetes deaths occur in developing countries, where four out of five people with diabetes reside (Aguiree et al., 2013).

Table 2 shows the number of people with diabetes in the IDF region, 2013. In 2013, the countries with the highest numbers of people aged 20 to 79 years with diabetes were: i) China (98.4 million); ii) India (65.1 million); iii) United States of America (U.S.) (24.4 million); iv) Brazil (11.9 million); v) Russian Federation (10.9 million); vi) Mexico (8.7 million); vii) Indonesia (8.5 million); viii) Germany (7.6 million); ix) Egypt (7.5 million); and x) Japan (7.2

million). The four main types of chronic diseases: CVD, cancers, CRD and diabetes account for 17.3, 7.6, 4.2 and 1.3 million deaths annually, respectively.

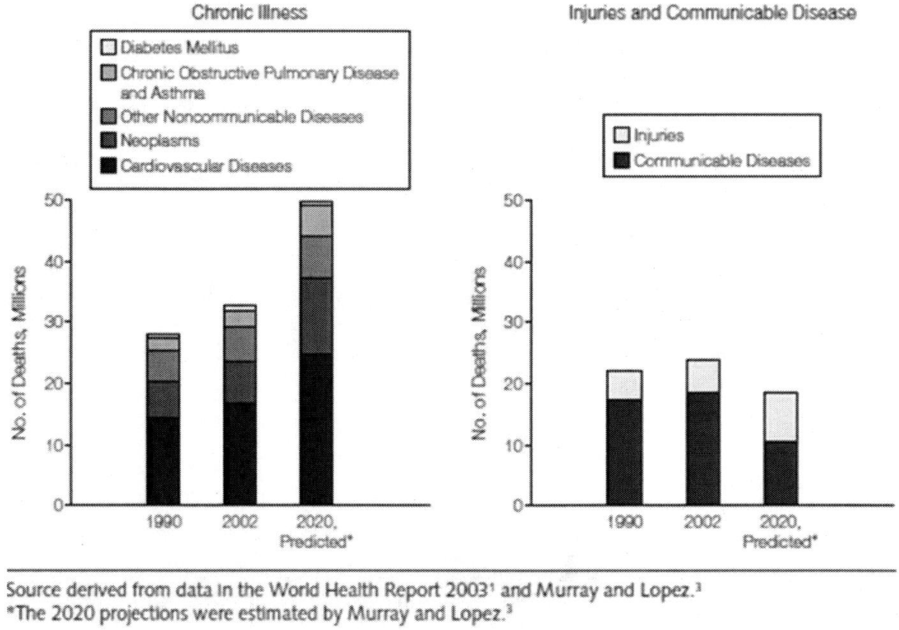

Source: Derived from data in the World Health Report 2003[1] and Murray and Lopez.[3]

* The 2020 projections were estimated by Murray and Lopez.[3]

Figure 7. Global Mortality from Chronic Diseases (Murray and Lopez, 2003).

Table 2. Number of people with diabetes, undiagnosed diabetes and projected increase in the IDF region, 2013

IDF Region	Number of People with Diabetes (in millions)	Percent Cases of Diabetes Undiagnosed, 2013	Projected Percent Increase in Cases, 2035
World	382	46	55.0
Western Pacific (WP)	138	54	46.0
South-East Asia (SEA)	72	49	70.6
Europe (EUR)	56	36	22.4
North America and Caribbean (NAC)	37	27	37.3
Middle East and North Africa (MENA)	35	48	96.2
South and Central America (SACA)	24	24	59.8
Africa (AFR)	20	62	109.1

Source: Aguiree et al. (2013).

Chronic Diseases and Developing Countries

Although the misnomer exists that the chronic disease epidemic is for affluent countries and only the elderly, the emerging data clearly show otherwise. The chronic disease epidemic is not exclusive to the developed countries; developing countries are disproportionally affected by chronic diseases. More than 80% of CVD deaths take place in developing countries, and occur almost equally in men and women (WHO, 2011a). Furthermore, the WHO reported that almost 80% of the 29 million deaths from chronic diseases occur in developing countries, with most of them occurring before the age of 60 (Lim et al., 2012). The World Bank has also indicated that chronic diseases increasingly threaten the health and economic security of developing countries.

Disturbingly, while the developing countries continue to have dramatic increases in chronic diseases, they also sustain high infectious disease burdens. As an example, in 2013 India had the second highest number of people with diabetes in the world (65.1 million), while at the same time 2.5 million Indian children die from infections annually (Aguiree et al., 2013). Correspondingly, in South Africa infectious and chronic diseases account for 28 and 25% of years of lives lost, respectively (Steyn et al., 2003). Overall, in Africa, infectious diseases are responsible for roughly 69% of deaths (Young et al., 2009). In Brazil, chronic diseases account for 72% of all deaths (Kulik 2013). In Russia, CVD is responsible for approximately 1.3 million deaths annually (Eberstadt, 2011), while 85% of the deaths in China are due to chronic diseases (Huang 2011).

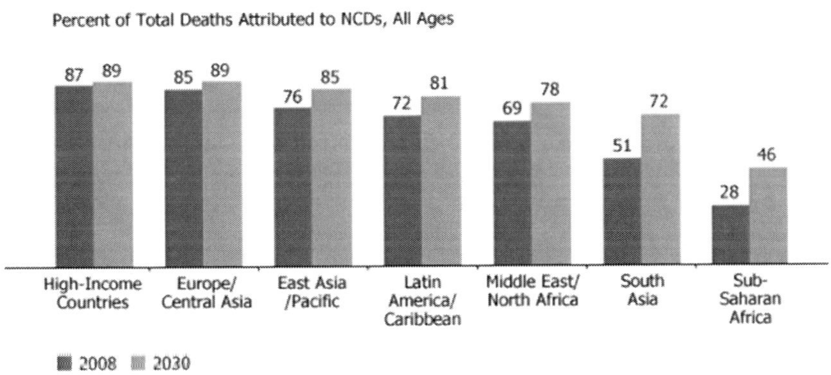

Figure 8. Chronic diseases account for a growing share of total deaths, especially in developing regions (Nikolic et al., 2011).

Over the next decade, Africa will experience the largest increases in death rates from CVD, cancer, diabetes and respiratory diseases (WHO, 2005). It is predicted that by 2030 in South Asia and Sub Saharan Africa, 21 and 18% of total deaths, respectively, would be attributed to chronic diseases (Figure 8). As compared to the developed countries, increases in deaths from chronic diseases are quite high in the developing countries. East Asia/Pacific, Latin America/Caribbean and Middle East/North Africa will have equally higher increases in chronic diseases death than the developed countries (Figure 8). The following examples demonstrate the seriousness of chronic diseases in the developing world. The information is taken from the World Health Organization's non-communicable disease (NCD) country profiles, 2014. For example, in Trinidad and Tobago, chronic diseases have been estimated to account for 80% of total deaths in 2012 (Table 3). In Morocco and the Bahamas, chronic diseases have been estimated to account for 75 and 72%, respectively, of all deaths (Table 3).

Table 3. Estimated percent of chronic disease deaths in selected developing countries (2012)

Available at: www.who.intlnmh/countries/sgp_en.pdf

Income Group	Country	Total Deaths	Chronic Disease Deaths (%)
High	Trinidad and Tobago	13,000	80
	Singapore	23,000	75
	Bahamas	2,200	72
Upper middle	Gabon	15,000	36
	Jamaica	20,000	79
Lower middle	Ghana	210,000	42
	India	9,816,000	60
	Morocco	206,000	75
Low income	Gambia	15,000	32
	Nepal	186,000	60
	Myanmar	441,000	59

Determinants of Chronic Diseases

This book defines determinants as influences, which affect an individual's ability to remain healthy, become ill, or injured. Normally, determinants can impact positively or negatively on chronic disease. In other words, determinants of chronic diseases could be either positive or negative. Positive determinants are described as protective, while those that are negative are referred to as risk factors. Several determinants of chronic diseases have been put forward in the literature. Urbanization, population aging, globalization of consumer markets and economic development are included are included in the list of underlying determinants (WHO, 2005).

Urbanization

Urbanization describes the process whereby there is a change in size, density, and heterogeneity of cities; it refers also to the gradual increase in the proportion of people living in urban areas (Vlahov and Galea, 2002; Godfrey and Julian, 2005). This could be a result of rural to urban migration or a natural population increase due to a decrease in death rates while birth rates remain high (UN, 2007). As of 2007, more than 50% of the world's populations live in urban areas. In developing countries, the population growth in urban areas has been extremely high, and is expected to continue increasing (Table 4).

The United Nations Human Settlements Program (UN-HABITAT) estimates that by 2050, 66% of people around the world will live in urban areas. It is expected that 50% of

Asia's population will live in urban areas by 2020, while Africa is likely to reach a 50% urbanization rate by 2035. By 2050, the world population is expected to rise to 9.3 billion (United Nations, 2011). The population residing in urban areas is projected to rise to 6.3 billion by 2050. It is projected that by 2050 urban dwellers will account for 86 and 67% of the population in the developed and developing countries, respectively (United Nations, 2011). People residing in urban areas are exposed to a double burden of communicable and chronic diseases (Moore et al., 2003; Stephan and Satterthwaite, 2008).

Table 4. Urban population size and growth by world region (WHO, 2009)

	Mid-year population (millions)				Growth rate (%)		
Region	1950	1975	2000	2030	1950-1975	1975-2000	2000-2030
Asia	244	592	137	2697	3.5	3.4	2.2
Africa	32	102	295	787	4.6	4.2	3.3
Europe	287	455	534	540	1.8	0.6	0.04
NAM[1]	70	198	391	608	4.2	2.7	1.5
LAC[2]	110	180	243	335	2.0	1.2	1.0
Ocean[3]	8	15	231	32	2.5	1.7	1.1

[1]North America; [2]Latin America and the Caribbean; [3]Oceania

There are advantages and disadvantages to urbanization. For example, urbanization provides more opportunities for things such as increased economic benefits, education openings and health care services. On the other hand, urbanization could be disadvantageous, for example, in South America urbanization has been accompanied by increased stress, lack of physical activity and poor diet, which all contribute to chronic disease risks (Avezum et al., 2009). Other studies from China and India have associated high prevalence of physical inactivity among women and men within urban communities (Anand et al., 2007; Ng et al., 2009).

According to Hope (1989) and Schuftan (1999), urbanization often exacerbates geographic and socioeconomic disparities in health within societies. For example, Ezzati et al. (2005) positively associated body mass index (BMI) and cholesterol levels with increases in urbanization and national income. Allender et al. (2010) examined the association between urban areas and chronic disease risk in Tamil Nadu, India. There was a positive association between urban areas and smoking, BMI, blood pressure and low physical activity among men; and increased BMI and low physical activity among women. Similarly, Allender et al. (2011) examined the relationship between *urbanicity* and chronic disease risk factors among Sri Lankan men and women. The researchers reported that among the men and women, '*urbanicity*' was positively associated with physical inactivity, high BMI and diabetes mellitus. Dahly and Adair (2007) found a positive, linear relationship between *urbanicity* and total caloric intake, and the percentage of dietary fat. It should be noted that there is a difference between urbanization and *urbanicity*. According to Vlahov and Galea (2002), *urbanicity* refers to the impact of residing in urban areas at a given time.

The following case study on urbanization and chronic disease in Southeast Asia is summarized from Angkurawaranon et al. (2014) to illustrate its effect. The authors reviewed articles for urban exposure and certain chronic diseases: seven for CVD; five for cancer; nine for chronic respiratory disease; and 16 for diabetes. The cross-sectional studies reviewed for urbanization and CVD were conducted in Vietnam, Myanmar, Malaysia, Thailand and

Indonesia (Ishine et al., 2005; Fitzpatrick et al., 2012; Myo et al., 1992; Wada et al., 2005a; Lim et al. 1991; Ishine et al., 2006; Wada et al., 2005b). The findings indicated that urban exposure was significantly associated with higher and lower odds ratio of stroke in studies from Malaysia and Vietnam, respectively (Fitzpatrick et al., 2012; Lim et al., 1991). Studies from Myanmar (Myo et al., 1992) and Malaysia (Lim et al., 1991) showed no evidence and strong evidence, respectively, for coronary heart disease. Urbanization was significantly associated with lower odds of rheumatic heart in Myanmar (Myo et al. 1992). A positive association was seen among urbanization, lung and osteogenic cancers, but an inverse relation was seen with oropharyngeal cancer (Bovill et al., 1975; Simarak et al., 1977). In Southeast Asia, urbanization was positively associated with diabetes and respiratory diseases in children.

Aging Population

The world population is increasing; the United Nations (UN) projections indicate that there will be roughly 2 billion more people by 2050 (Figure 9). In 2025, 2050 and 2100, the world population is projected to stand at 8.1, 9.6 and 10.9 billion, respectively. All the population increases are predicted to impact developing countries profoundly, with minimal changes in the developed countries (United Nations Population Division, 2013). For example, the overall increase between 2013 and 2050 is projected to take place in Africa, India, Pakistan, Philippines and the U.S. (United Nations Population Division, 2013).

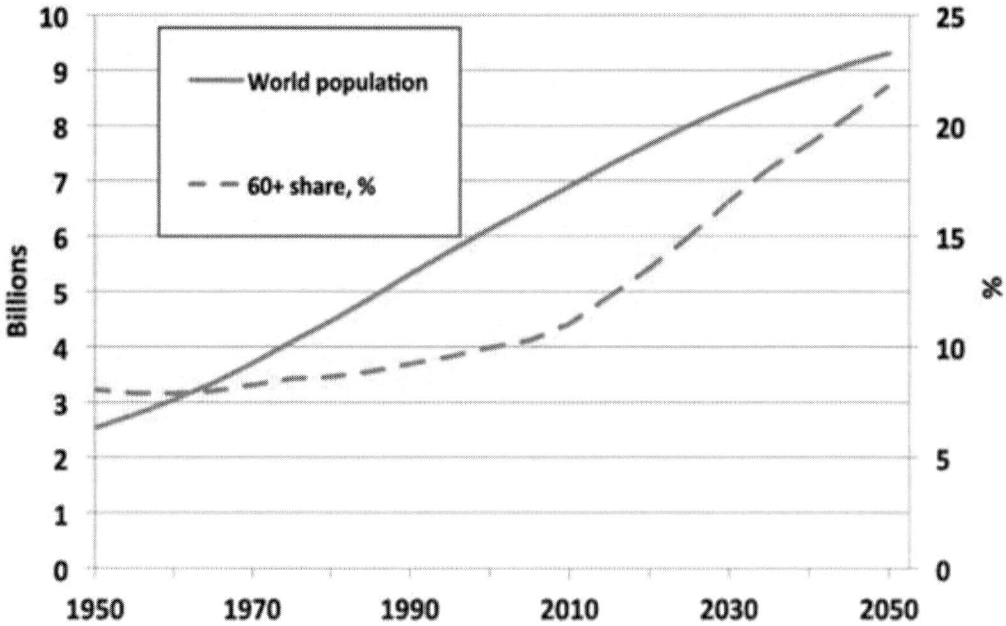

Figure 9. The world population is growing and getting older (United Nations Population Division, 2011).

Population aging allows more people to live to the age when chronic diseases become manifest. Population aging occurs when the birth rate exceeds the death rate and the number of individuals living on the planet increases (United Nations Population Division, 2013). The global trend reflects that persons 60 years and above are the most rapid growing group. In developing countries, 9% of the population is above age 60, and this proportion will more than double by 2050 and triple in 2100 (United Nations Population Division, 2013). Also, in developing countries, the annual population growth will be 2.9% before 2050 and 0.9% between 2050 and 2100 (United Nations Population Division, 2013). The rates are lower in the developed world (Figure 10). Additionally, the number of persons older than 80 years is expected to increase seven-fold by 2100 (assets.aarp.org).

The world's elderly population, more prone to chronic diseases is growing. Chronic diseases disproportionately affect people 65 years and over, therefore the incidence of these diseases is expected to increase in the future. Increasing prevalence of the key risk factors will also contribute to the urgency, particularly as globalization and urbanization take greater hold in the developing world. The rates of heart disease, hypertension, and cancer are all higher in older age cohorts. The risk for heart disease is three times higher in someone 75 years and older than in a person ages 50 to 64 years (assets.aarp.org). Similarly, the risk of hypertension is 66% higher for those 74 to 84 years old than for those 50 to 64 years old. Interestingly, those older than 85 years are not significantly sicker than those ages 75 to 84 years (assets.aarp.org). The risk of having five or more chronic conditions rises to 21% for those 85 years and over versus 8% for those ages 50 to 64 years (assets.aarp.org).

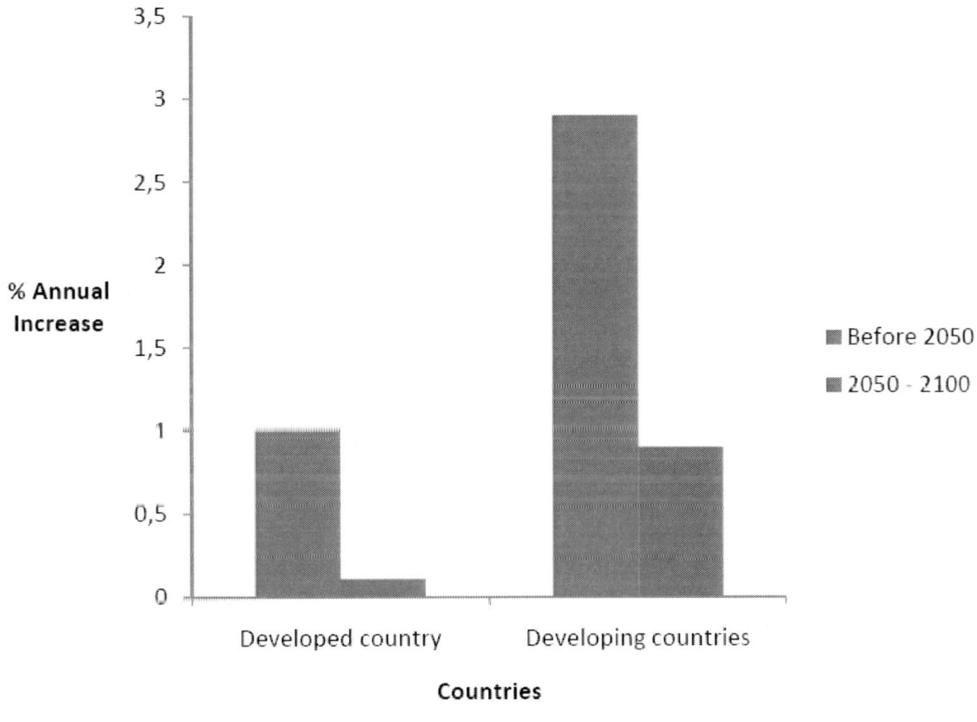

Figure 10. World population growth in the developed and developing world 2050-2100. Available at: assets.aarp.org.

Globalization

Globalization is a process of interaction and integration among the people, companies, and governments of different nations. The process is usually propelled by international trade and investment facilitated by information technology. The concept of globalization is archaic. For example, subsequent to the industrial revolution in England and Europe, millions of meters of cotton were exported to developing countries (Hobsbawn 1996). Globalization has effects on environment, culture, political systems, economic development, and human physical well-being in societies universally. Stuckler (2008) has used globalization as a theoretical framework for better understanding of the current and future rising risk of chronic disease, especially in developing countries.

Three structural aspects of globalization, namely, economic flows, economic growth, and technological change have been used by Stuckler (2008) to demonstrate the influence of globalization on chronic disease. In terms of economic flows, Stuckler (2008) cited increased global interconnectivity as facilitating the free flow of goods, resources and services across countries. In relating these economic flows to behavioral risks, the author pointed out that these flows mainly promote easily transported processed and pre-packaged items such as sugary beverages and cigarettes. Stuckler (2008) further postulated that economic growth increased income levels in populations, which in turn impact upon dietary and consumption patterns. In developed countries, people tend to purchase more healthy foods and increase physical activity as their income levels rise (Stucker, 2008). However, the opposite appears to be true in population's risk of chronic diseases. Stuckler (2008) concluded that: i) globalization leads to greater inter-country dietary dependence; ii) foreign direct investment in foods developing countries (Drewnowski and Darmon 2005). As societies advance technologically, labor shifts occur and workplaces become more sedentary. Work becomes more centralized as technologies and service industries grow, for example, the call centers in India. Such work opportunities increase people's movement from rural to urban settings. It should be noted that urban settings in developing countries have limited opportunities for physical activity. Furthermore, as more women enter the workforce (in part due to the technological advances), food consumption outside the home increases.

Stuckler (2008) stated that economic flows have improved the accessibility of behavioral risks; the social changes accompanying economic growth have encouraged their adoption; and technological change has created incentives for people to become more physically inactive and consume more meals outside the home. Stuckler (2008) argued that all the aforementioned factors combined, increases beverages in developing countries favoring less healthy products; iii) transnational companies' marketing strategies influence/change the sensory preferences of individuals in developing countries as incomes rise; and iv) technological change speeds up all these processes, encourages more sedentary lifestyles, and shifts the locus of food consumption away from the home. Globalization through more interdependent worldwide trade relationships, especially regarding food supplies has, and will continue to contribute to the rising risk of chronic disease and mortality in the developing world.

All in all, in developing countries, urbanization, population-aging and globalization act together to increase exposure to common modifiable risk factors for chronic diseases including: unhealthy diets, physical inactivity, tobacco use and harmful use of alcohol.

Risk Factors for Chronic Disease

What Are the Risk Factors for Chronic Diseases?

The risk factors for chronic diseases are well established. A small set of common risk factors are responsible for most of the main chronic diseases. In both males and females, the major risk factors are unhealthy diet, physical inactivity, and tobacco use, which are all modifiable (WHO, 2005). They are manifested through the intermediate risk factors of raised blood pressure, raised glucose levels, abnormal blood lipids, overweight and obesity (Table 5). The major modifiable risk factors, in conjunction with the non-modifiable risk factors of age and heredity explain the majority of new events of heart disease, stroke, chronic respiratory diseases and some important cancers (Table 5). The relationship between the major modifiable risk factors and the main chronic diseases is similar in all regions of the world.

Table 5. Risk factors for chronic diseases (WHO, 2005)

UNDERLYING SOCIOECONOMIC, CULTURAL, POLITICAL AND ENVIRONMENTAL DETERMINANTS	COMMON MODIFIABLE RISK FACTORS	INTERMEDIATE RISK FACTORS	MAIN CHRONIC DISEASES
Globalization	Unhealthy diet	Raised blood pressure	Cardiovascular diseases
Urbanization	Physical inactivity	Raised blood glucose	Cancer
Population aging	Tobacco use	Abnormal blood lipids	Chronic respiratory diseases
	NON-MODIFIABLE RISK FACTORS	Overweight/obesity	Diabetes
	Age		
	Heredity		

Several other risk factors, which account for a smaller proportion of chronic diseases have been, identified (WHO, 2005). Detrimental alcohol use is a significant provider to the global burden of disease; however, its association with chronic disease has not been clearly elucidated. Other risk factors for chronic disease include: i) infectious agents, which are responsible for cervical and liver cancers; ii) some environmental factors, such as air pollution, which contribute to an array of chronic diseases, such as asthma and other chronic respiratory diseases; and iii) psychosocial and genetic factors (WHO, 2005).

According to WHO (2005), there is now extensive evidence from many countries that conditions *in utero* and in early childhood influence health in adult life. For example, it is now known that there is a relationship between low birth weight and increased rates of high blood pressure, heart disease, stroke and diabetes. Aging is also a critical marker for the accrual of modifiable risks for chronic disease, as the impact of risk factors increases during the progression of life (Table 5). The underlying determinants of chronic diseases mentioned earlier are reflective of the main influences compelling social, economic and cultural change. It is also well known that chronic diseases and poverty are highly interconnected (WHO, 2005). Figure 11 demonstrates how chronic diseases contribute to poverty and vice versa.

In most countries, the poorest people are at highest risk of developing chronic diseases and dying prematurely from them. Several reasons have been advanced to explain why the chronic disease burden is concentrated among the poor. To list a few, the poor are more vulnerable to chronic diseases because of: i) material deprivation and psychosocial stress; ii) higher levels of risk behavior; iii) unhealthy living conditions; and iv) limited access to good-quality health care (WHO, 2005). Quoting directly from WHO (2011), "chronic diseases and poverty create a vicious cycle whereby poverty exposes people to behavioral risk factors for chronic diseases and, in turn, the resulting chronic diseases may become an important driver to the downward spiral that leads families towards poverty."

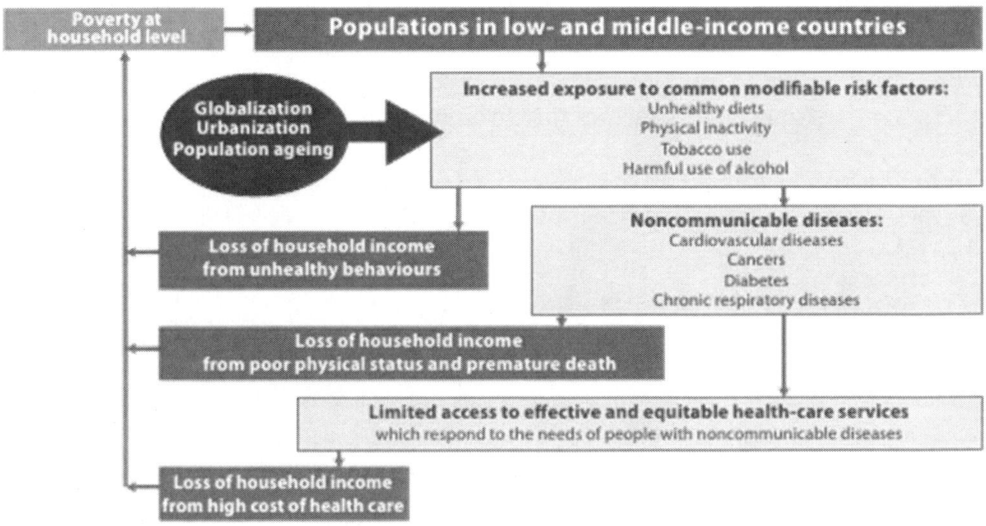

Figure 11. Poverty-chronic disease relationship (WHO, 2010). Global status report on NCDs 2010. Available at: http://www.globalissues.org; accessed 08/24/2015.

Nutrition Transition

The unparalleled rise in chronic diseases globally has been associated with the phenomenon of nutrition transition (Di Rocco and Cuvi, 2014). Several definitions have been put forth for nutrition transition. Using the definition given by Popkin et al. (2001), nutrition transition is characterized by a shift away from monotonous diets of varying nutritional quality (based on indigenous grains or starchy roots, locally grown legumes, other vegetables and fruits, and limited foods of animal origin) toward more varied diets that include processed food, higher intakes of animal source foods, sugar, fat, and oftentimes harmful alcohol consumption (Popkin, Horton & Kim 2001). These factors are exacerbated by physical inactivity resulting in rapid increases in overweight and obesity.

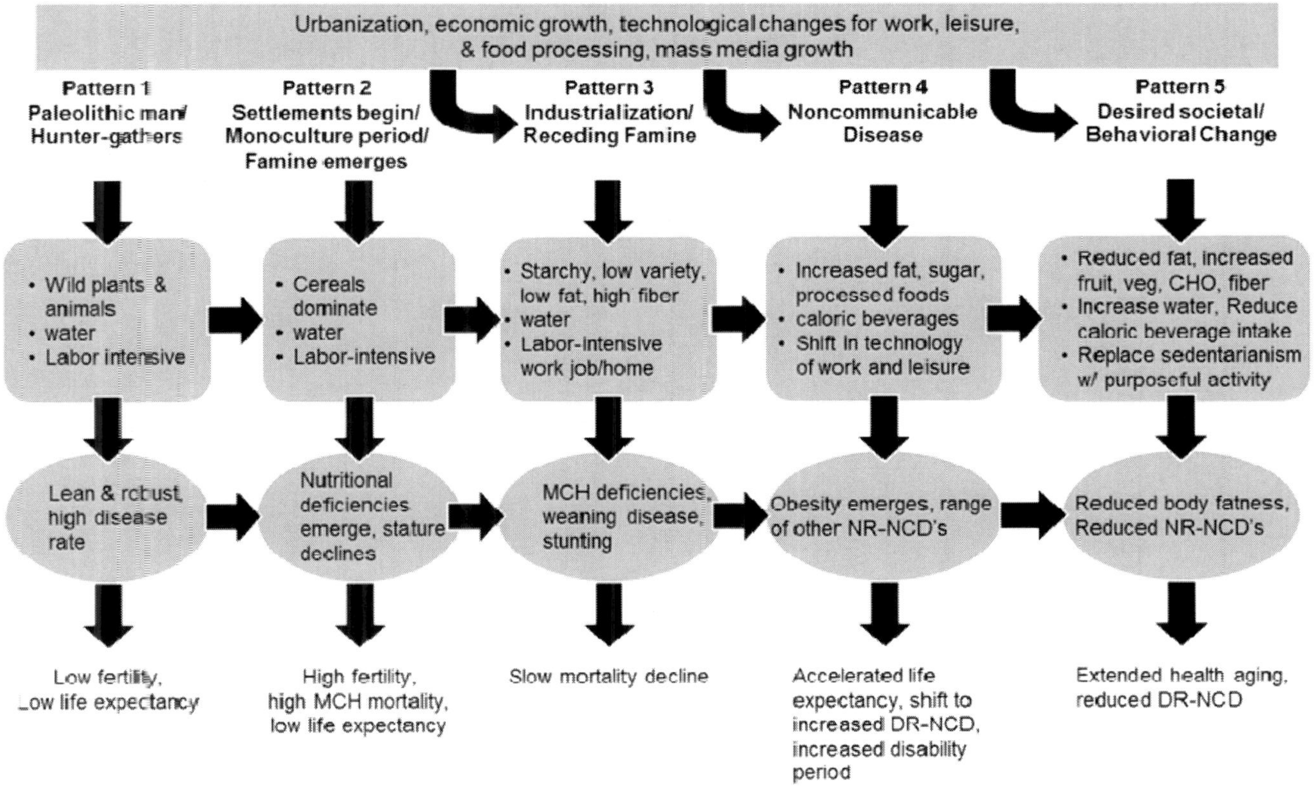

Figure 12. The stages of nutrition transition (Popkin, 2002).

Doak and Popkin (2008) and Cabellero (2005) stated that nutrition transition is characterized by the prevalence of overweight/obesity surpassing malnutrition, and an increase in deaths from chronic diseases in developing countries. Popkin and Gordon-Larsen (2004) simply defined nutrition transition as being representative of a society's switch in dietary consumption and physical activity, which results from globalization, epidemiological and demographic transitions. Popkin (2002) described the stages of nutrition transition as shown in Figure 12. According to Popkin (2001) three distinct stages of nutrition transition include: i) early stage of stage 1 in which under-nutrition rates are high, and overweight and obesity are just starting to emerge; ii) in double burden or stage 2, the rates of under-nutrition and overweight/obesity are both high; and iii) the completed transition or stage 3 has low prevalence of under-nutrition, but high prevalence of overweight/obesity.

Nutrition transition has also been defined as an overall global shift towards diets high in fat, sugar and salt, and low in fresh fruits, vegetables and fiber (Popkin, 2003; Di Rocco and Cuvi, 2014). Subsequent to the industrial revolution, there was a shift in the methods of food production, processing, storage, and distribution (WHO, 2002a). Additionally, economic development, technological advances and modern marketing techniques have transformed dietary preferences leading to major changes in consumption patterns of most populations across the world. Such changes in food consumption pattern promote an array of diet-related chronic diseases.

The nutrition transition first started in the developed world and then occurred very rapidly in the developing countries. For example, there was an estimated 5 to10 fold increase in the per person consumption of fat and refined carbohydrates in England over the past two centuries, while the consumption of fiber-rich grains decreased dramatically (WHO, 2002a). There is much inter- and intra- country variation in rate of, and the factors influencing the transition (Popkin 2002). Popkin (2003) aligns the nutrition transition with three distinct shifts: i) demographic shift from high to low rates of fertility, and mortality associated with consumption of diets high in fat, sugar and salt, and low in fresh fruits, vegetables and fiber; ii) epidemiological shift from high incidence of communicable diseases to high incidence of chronic diseases; and iii) shift in the consciousness and behavior of individuals marked by healthier diet-related habits and efforts to prevent chronic diseases. For example, developing countries such as Brazil, Chile, Ecuador, Mexico, Peru, and the Dominican Republic are deemed to be experiencing the nutrition transition. Since 2000, these countries have undergone increases in: obesity, dietary fat intake and chronic disease mortality along with declining incidence of infant mortality and stunting (Abrahams et al., 2011; Albala et al., 2001; Ford and Mokdad, 2008; Uauy et al; 2001; Kain et al., 2003; Rojas-Martínez et al., 2012; Bonvecchio et al., 2009; Rivera, 2009).

Factors which impact the nutrition transition include high urbanization rates, globalization, economic development, population aging, and biological factors. To reiterate, urbanization is associated with high physical inactivity, increased overweight and obesity (Henry et al., 2001; Yamauchi et al., 2001; Mokhtar et al., 2001). Urban populations tend to be more dependent on processed, store-bought foods as compared to their rural counterparts (Solomons 1995). It follows that salt and simple sugar intakes will increase among urban populations (Popkin 2002). Also, urbanization leads to consumption of new types and more refined grains (Drewnowski and Popkin, 1997). For example, store-bought bread is readily accessible, and is rapidly replacing traditional staples in many developing countries, primarily in urban settings. According to Popkin (2002), a shift from 25 to 75% urban population in very low-income countries would be associated with a 4% increased energy intake from fat and a 12% of energy intake from sweeteners.

Globalization has been linked to greater availability of inexpensive dietary fat and rapid changes in social, cultural and sensory preferences. The changeover in staple consumption usually comes with increased fat (especially saturated fat) intake, as well as sugar and other refined carbohydrates (Solomons 1995). The increased fat intake results, not from the staple per se, but rather from the types of accompaniment eaten with the staple. For example, many sauces that are eaten with rice, roots and tubers are much less fatty than cheeses, processed meat, meat products (like sausages) and fat spreads that are eaten with bread (Popkins 2002). In the globalization process, saturated fats, trans- fatty acids, and inexpensive vegetable oils become more accessible to populations.

Further, globalization of food production directly impacts the nutrition transition. To illustrate, technological advances allow for mass production, which reduces the price of selected food items; and global distribution and marketing expedite the introduction of processed foods to a wide range of countries. It should be pointed out that by and large, the economic growth of developed countries is usually dependent on expansion of markets into developing countries (Cabellero and Popkin, 2002). Sequentially, a high percentage of global food production will be driven by the demands of developing country mainly because of population growth (Cabellero and Popkin, 2002).

To briefly summarize the chapter, the prevalence of chronic diseases is expected to rise by over 20% in Africa and South-East Asia by 2020. The developing countries are disproportionally affected by chronic diseases. Almost 80% of deaths from chronic diseases now occur in developing countries. Unless urgent action is taken, 41 and 55 million people will die of a chronic disease in 2015 and 2030, respectively. It is predicted that by 2030 in South Asia and Sub Saharan Africa, 21 and 18% of total deaths, respectively, would be attributed to chronic diseases. The major determinants of chronic diseases are urbanization, aging population and globalization, these are all happening at a rate in the developing world. The major risk factors for chronic diseases are unhealthy diet, physical inactivity, and tobacco use, which are all modifiable. Individuals are more susceptible to these risk factors in situations where there is growing urbanization and globalization as experienced in many developing countries. The unparalleled rise in chronic diseases globally has been associated with the phenomenon of nutrition transition, which again is linked to high urbanization rates, and aging population among other things.

Economic Burden of Chronic Diseases

Magnitude of the Problem

Chronic diseases are placing an enormous burden on countries worldwide. The economic impact might actually be much worse in developing countries, but the data are still scarce. Using diabetes to illustrate, it is interesting to note that only 20% of global health expenditure was spent on diabetes in the developing countries, where 80% of people with diabetes live (IDF, 2013). The U.S. spent US$239 billion of its health dollars on diabetes, or 36% of global health expenditure. Meanwhile, China, the country with the most people living with diabetes, spent just US$38 billion, less than 7% of the global total. The combined spending of the top three countries, the U.S., Germany and China, was equivalent to more than 50% of all global health expenditure on diabetes in 2013. Norway spent an average of US$ 10,368 on diabetes healthcare per person with diabetes, while countries such as Somalia and Eritrea spent less than US$30 (IDF, 2013).

Annual deaths attributable to diabetes are probably as high as 3 million with more than 80% occurring in developing countries. Increasing prevalence of chronic diseases is a major contributor for rapid rise in healthcare cost in developing countries since the last decade. Worldwide estimates suggest that the annual direct medical cost for diabetes in total is at least US$129 billion and may be as high as US$241 billion, or 2.5 to 15.0% of global annual healthcare budget. It was also estimated that there will be almost 50% increase in direct healthcare costs associated with diabetes from US$286 billion in 2003 to US$396 billion in 2025 (Zawiah 2007).

Lower middle-income countries (LMIC) shown in Table 1 account for 84 and 83% of the world's population and chronic disease, respectively, as measured by disability adjusted life years (DALYs) (World Economic Forum, Harvard School of Public Health, 2011). The projections shown in Table 6 reveal that more than $7 trillion will be lost from the four major chronic diseases in LMIC between 2011 to 2025; averaging roughly US$500 bn. annually (World Economic Forum, Harvard School of Public Health, 2011). In 2010, for low- and middle- income countries, the annual loss of roughly US$ 500 billion was equal to 4% of their gross domestic product (GDP) (World Economic Forum, Harvard School of Public Health, 2011). To further illustrate, on an individual basis, this yearly loss averages US$ 25, 50 and 139 for low-, middle- and upper middle- income countries, respectively. Stuckler et al. (2010) concluded that for every 10% rise in mortality from chronic conditions, the yearly economic growth of a country is estimated to be reduced by 0.5 percentage points.

Table 6. Economic burden of chronic diseases, 2011-2025 (trillions of US$ in 2008)

Country Income Group	Diabetes	CVD*	Respiratory Diseases	Cancer	Total
Upper middle	0.31	2.52	1.09	1.20	5.12
Lower middle	0.09	1.07	0.44	0.26	1.85
Low income	0.02	0.17	0.06	0.05	0.31
Total of low and middle	0.42	3.76	1.59	1.51	7.28

*Cardiovascular diseases.
World Economic Forum, Harvard School of Public Health, 2011.

Approaches for Measuring the Economic Burden

Three alternative approaches for measuring the economic burden of chronic diseases such as diabetes have been presented in the literature. These approaches, willingness-to-pay, cost-of-illness and macroeconomic/production function are discussed elsewhere (Kirigia et al., 2000; Kirigia et al., 2003; Kirigia et al., 2004). The conceptual framework of the economic burden of diabetes is presented to illustrate how it works for chronic diseases (Figure 13).

Using the cost-of-illness approach described by Kirigia et al. (2009), the economic burden of diabetes comprises of direct, indirect and intangible costs.

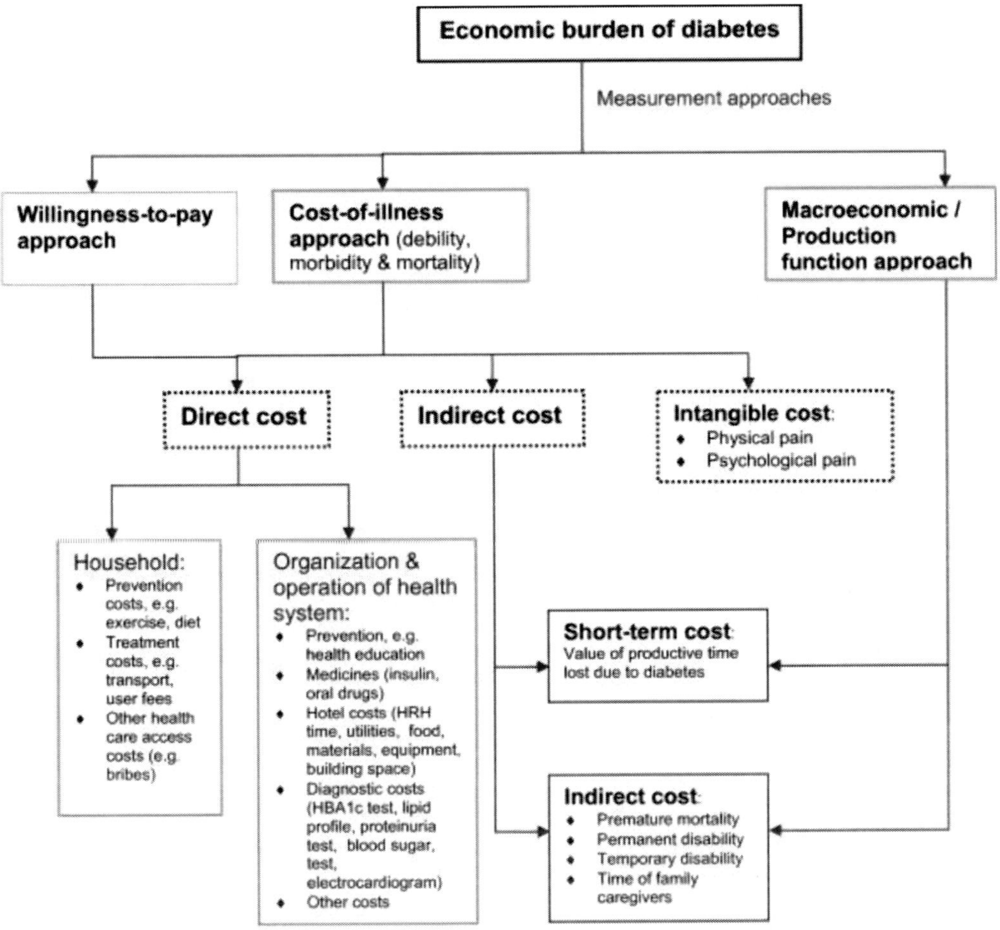

Figure 13. Conceptual framework of the economic burden of diabetes (Kirigia *et al.,* 2009).

Cost-of-Illness

Indirect Costs (Costs of Lost Production)

Recent studies have indicated that chronic diseases will cost the world economy US$47 trillion in direct healthcare costs, lost output and untimely death over the next two decades (NCD Alliance, 2010). Currently, the developed countries bear the largest economic burden of chronic diseases. However, developing countries are expected to carry the larger economic burden by the next decade and a half (Jha et al., 2012). The global economic effects of chronic disease will result in long-term economic impacts on labor supply, capital accumulation and GDP, especially in developing countries (Mayer-Foulkes, 2011; Nikolic et al., 2011).

Table 7. Global economic burden of chronic diseases, 2011-2030 based on the EPIC model

Country income group	Share of global economic loss from chronic disease 2010	Share of global population 2010	Share of global mortality 2008	Share of global income (constant US$ 2,000)	Total loss	CVD	Cancers	CRD	Diabetes	Mental Illness
Low (L)	0.02	0.12	0.43	0.01	0.9	0.3	0.1	0.1	0.0	0.3
Lower-middle (LM)	0.12	0.37	0.32	0.05	5.4	2.0	0.5	0.9	0.2	1.9
Upper middle (UM)	0.32	0.36	0.10	0.19	14.9	4.8	2.3	2.2	0.6	5.1
High	0.55	0.16	0.14	0.75	25.5	8.5	5.4	1.6	1.0	9.0
L + LM + UM	0.45	0.84	0.85	0.25	21.2	7.1	2.9	3.2	0.8	7.3
World					**46.7**	**15.6**	**8.3**	**4.8**	**1.7**	**16.3**

CVD – cardiovascular disease; CRD – chronic respiratory disease (Jha et al., 2012).

According to Fuster and Kelly (2010), the economic consequence of CVD and other chronic diseases such as diabetes is enormous for developing countries. As an example, the global economic cost of new cancer cases in 2009 was US$286 billion (Bloom et al., 2011). In China, the annual direct medical costs of obesity-related diabetes, CHD and stroke was estimated at US$3 billion (Fuster and Kelly, 2010). In Brazil, 72% of all deaths are caused by chronic diseases (Schmidt et al., 2011).

The annual economic burden for treatment and lost productivity from five chronic diseases in Brazil was estimated at US$72 billion (Fuster and Kelly (2010). In South Africa, the state spends US$19,500 annually treating a single patient on dialysis (IRIN, 2013).

The presence and growing prevalence of chronic diseases in developing countries will continue to present primary stumbling blocks to economic growth (Kulic, 2013). In this book, the intent of the estimates described for each disease is to share with readers the extent of costs for each illness. They are certainly not intended to be used as direct comparisons for the cost of each disease category, and how they rank against each other.

Projections from Jha et al. (2012) indicate that the total lost output from five chronic diseases between 2011 and 2030 will be US$47 trillion (Table 7). This total loss is indicative of an annual 5% of global GDP in 2010 according to Jha et al. (2012). Upon closer examination of Table 7, it can be seen that developing countries will share 45% of the economic losses from chronic diseases, even though they account for only 25% of the global income.

The U.S. workforce illness costs $576 billion annually from sick days to workers' compensation. According to the Integrated Benefits Institute (2014), poor health costs the U.S. economy $576 bn. annually, of which 39% is from lost productivity. Chronic conditions like diabetes, heart disease or depression can trigger absenteeism, presenteeism, disability and workers compensation claims.

Figure 14 shows an example of lost economic output associated with seven common chronic health problems. The average annual days lost by workers with chronic diseases are shown in Figure 15. Workers with chronic conditions were more likely to miss work than peers without a chronic disease. Both older and younger workers with more than one chronic disease were more likely to miss more work days than those with one or no chronic disease (Figure 14). For those with one chronic disease, the older workers missed more work days than the younger ones (Figure 14).

Sick leave places a substantial economic burden in societies where employees receive sick leave benefits (Taimela et al., 2007). The presence of chronic disease has been associated with increased sick leave, which has been shown to be more prevalent in older people (De Klerk, 2000). Donders et al. (2012) reported that with employees <36 and 55 + years of age, the 55+ employees had a decreased risk of frequent sick leave, and an elevated risk of prolonged sick leave.

The researchers inferred that the presence of chronic disease partially explained the sick leave in the two older groups. Their findings supported previous reports that chronic diseases are a major cause of long-term sickness, absence and job loss (Detaille et al., 2009).

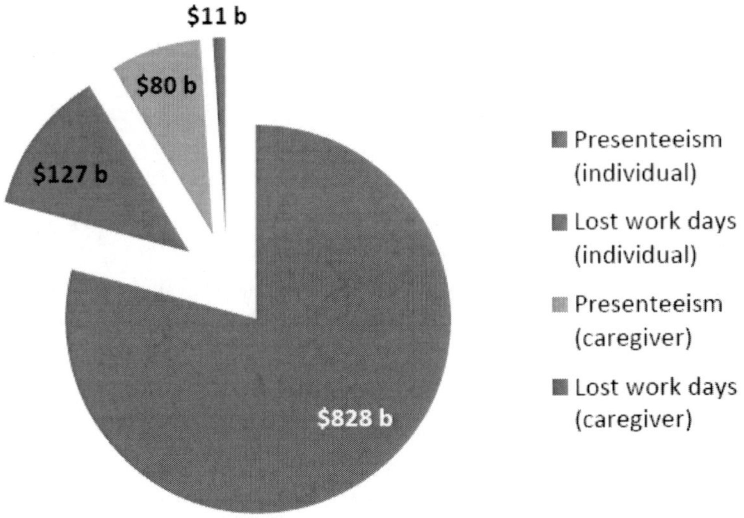

Figure 14. Lost economic output for common chronic health problems (DeVol et al., 2007).

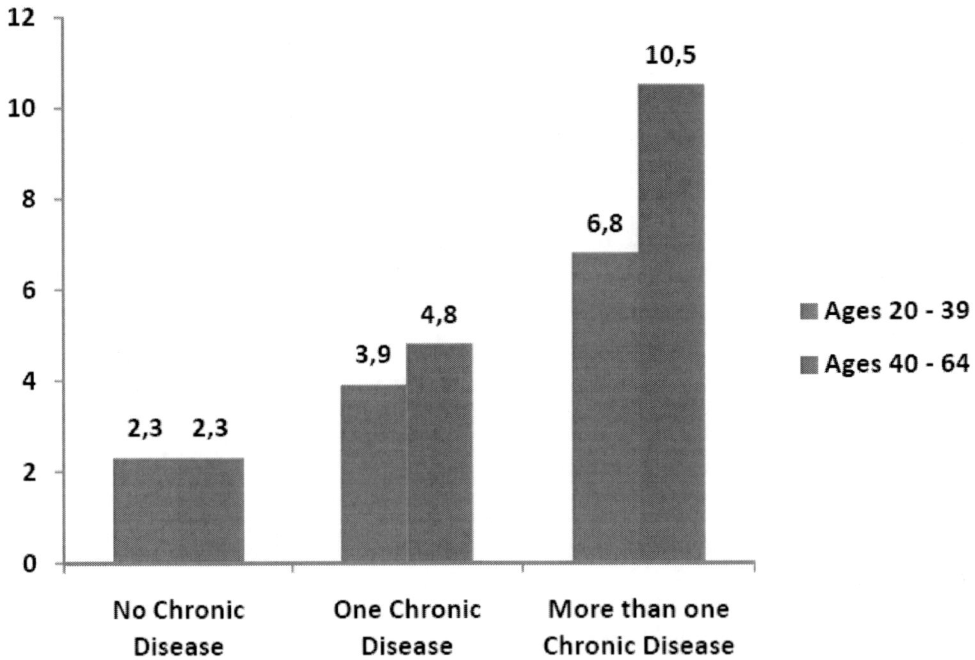

Figure 15. Average annual days lost by workers with chronic condition (U.S. Chamber of Commerce and Partnership for Prevention, 2007).

Cost-of-Illness

Some of the major elements of direct cost-of-illness (COI), actual expenditure are shown in Figure 16. COI data are detailed elsewhere by Jha et al. (2012), who presented estimates for individual chronic diseases. For example, global new cancer cases of 13.3 million in 2010 were estimated to cost US$290 billion. Further breakdowns revealed that medical costs, non-medical costs, and income losses accounted for US$154, 67 and 69 billion, respectively. Bloom et al. (2011) further predicted that there will be roughly 1.5 time increase in this number by year 2030.

Global estimates for CVD in 2010 were US$863 billion, which is projected to increase to US$1,044 billion in 2030. Roughly 55 and 45% of the US$863 billion were due to direct healthcare costs, absenteeism, presenteeism and premature death (Bloom et al., 2011). A report from the World Economic Forum and the Harvard School of Public Health indicated that developing countries will share the growing global cost of COPD (Bloom et al., 2011). In 2010, the global cost of COPD was US$2.1 trillion with a predicted increase to US$4.8 trillion in 2030; roughly 50% of all global costs will be in the developing countries (Bloom et al., 2011). In 2009, the total cost for new cancer cases was 647, 8,209 and 8,945 million for lower, middle and upper-income countries, respectively (Beaulieu et al., 2009). The total cost included medical, non-medical and productivity losses. The examples in this section focus primarily on one of the major chronic diseases, diabetes, for illustrative purposes.

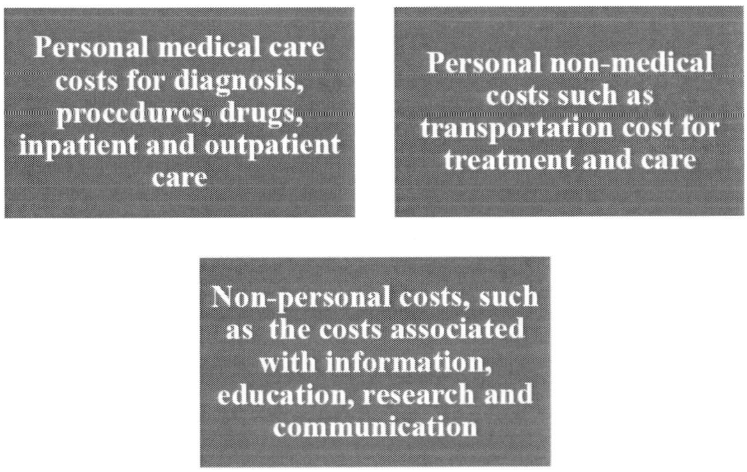

Figure 16. Some major elements of direct cost-of-illness (COI) (Bloom et al., 2011).

For diabetes, the global cost was approximately US$500 billion (bn.) in 2010 with an expected increase to US$745 bn. by 2030; the greatest burden will occur in the developing world (Bloom et al., 2011). Globally, health spending on diabetes accounted for 10.8% of total health expenditure 2013 (IDF, 2013). In 2013, global health spending to treat and manage complications from diabetes amounted to roughly US$548 bn.; this number is estimated to surpass US$627 bn. by 2035 (IDF, 2013). A projected average of US$1,437 per person was spent globally on treatment and management of diabetes in 2013 (IDF, 2013).

Barcelo et al. (2003) reported that the total costs due to diabetes for Venezuela and Barbados were 1.8 and 5.9% of GDP, respectively. Medical costs of diabetes care for patients visiting private facilities were between 15 and 25% of household income in India (Shobhana et al., 2000). In Saudi Arabia, people diagnosed with diabetes, had medical healthcare expenditures that were 10 times higher (US$3,686 versus $380) than those without diabetes (Alhowaish, 2013). Islam and Azad (2014) reported the mean yearly cost of care for diabetes was US$314 in Bangladesh; with direct and indirect costs of US$283 and 37, respectively. Afroz (2012) indicated that the mean yearly cost of diabetes care per patient in outpatient departments of tertiary care facility in Bangladesh was US$ 313. Using this estimate, the total yearly burden for the estimated 9.5 million diabetic patients in the country will be US$2973.5 million.

In Mexico, the average annual cost per diabetic patient was US$708; the total annual cost of diabetics was US$2,618,000, which is 15.5 and 0.8% of health spending and GDP, respectively (Table 8). It has been predicted that by 2020, the Canadian economy will lose $11 bn. per year due to mortality of diabetes patients. Additionally, long-term care costs are expected to increase from $1 bn. to $2.7 bn. annually over that time period for diabetes patients (Canadian Diabetes Association, 2009). According to Abdulganiyu and Fola (2014), the annual national cost of illness for diabetes mellitus in Nigeria, may be about US$1,521,014.644; while the average annual cost of illness was roughly US$319, about 88% of the yearly per capita income. The cost of type 2 diabetes for other countries is shown in Table 8.

In Jamaica, 59% of households affected with chronic disease underwent financial difficulties (Henry-Lee and Yearwood, 1999). Similarly, in Burkina Faso, financial difficulties increased by 50% in households touched by chronic disease (Su et al., 2006). In Europe, chronic disease, especially of a husband, raised the probability of premature retirement (Suhrcke 2006). Chronic disease resulted in 5.6% lower median per-person income in Russia (Mayer-Foulkes 2011).

Table 8. Cost of type 2 diabetes in selected developing countries

Country	Author	Average Medical Cost
Pakistan	Khowaja et al., 2007	Mean direct cost per visit, no co-morbidity was US$14.31. One or more co-morbidities was US$20.7
Thailand	Riewpaiboon et al., 2007	Average direct medical cost per year US$205.95 both type 1 and type 2 diabetes
	Chatterjee et al., 2011	Total cost of illness of diabetes for 475 study participants was estimated at US$ 418,696 for the financial year 2008. 23% was Direct medical, direct non-medical and indirect costs were 23, 40 and 37%, respectively. The mean cost of illness per diabetic patient was US$881.47 in 2008, which was 21% of per capita GDP of Thailand. Existence of complications increased the cost substantially. Cost of informal care contributed 28% of total cost of illness of diabetes, thus also affecting family members, friends, neighbors etc.
Sudan	Elravah-Eliadarous, 2007	Direct median cost per year - US$175
Taiwan	Wu-Chang et al., 2001	Medical cost per patient year annual-US$26,988 Outpatient - US$22,311; inpatient - US$4,677
Mexico	Villareal-Rios, 2000	Total annual cost US$ 2,618,00, 15.5% of health spending and 0.79% of GDP; annual cost per diabetic patient was US$708
Bangladesh	Islam and Azad, 2014	Annual cost US$314 (direct cost US$238 and indirect US$37)
India	Islam and Azad, 2014	Annual direct cost per patient US$152.58

Cancer is one of the most costly diseases in the U.S. The latest estimates from the National Institutes of Health (NIH) have revealed that the overall economic costs of cancer in 2009 were $216.6 and $130.0 bn. for direct and indirect costs, respectively (ACS, 2014). It should be noted that the 2009 cost is much higher than the combined NIH and National Cancer Institute (NCI) budgets for fiscal year 2014. Globally, in 2009, 12.9 million new cancer cases were diagnosed and the estimated cost was $286 bn. (Stewart and Wild, 2015). In 2010, the global cost for 13.3 million newly diagnosed cancer cases was estimated at $290 to $300 billion (http://www.bloomberg.com). The projected 21.5 million new cases for 2030 are expected to cost $458 bn. (http://www.bloomberg.com).

The cumulative global cost for dialysis and transplantation from kidney disease over the next decade is predicted to exceed US$ 1 trillion. This economic burden could strain healthcare budgets in developed countries. The economic burden for developing countries is particularly severe, partly because CKD generally occurs at a younger age (Jha et al., 2013). For example, in Guatemala, 40% of patients receiving RRT are under 40. Of the individuals receiving renal replacement therapy (RRT), more than 80% reside in the developed world. RRT is mostly unaffordable in developing countries. In countries such as India and Pakistan, less than 10% of all patients who need it receive any kind of RRT and in many African countries there is little or no access to RRT. Table 9 represents examples of the cost of kidney disease in some developed and developing countries.

Table 9. Examples of the cost of kidney disease in some developed and developing countries

Year	Country	Type of kidney disease	Annual cost	Estimated annual cost by 2020
	Australia	End stage (ESKD)		AUS$12 billion
1996	Japan	ESKD	4% of total healthcare budget	
2000-2001	Australia	Chronic kidney disease (CKD)	AU$647 million	
2004	South Korea	ESKD	3.24% of national health expenditure	
2007	U.S.	CKD	Medicare >US$60 bn. (27% total Medicare budget)	
2009-2010	United Kingdom	CKD	£1.44 - 1.45 bn.	
	Nigeria	ESKD	US$100/session for hemodialysis	
	India	ESKD	US$20 - 60/session for hemodialysis	
Annual	Uruguay	ESKD	US$23 million (30% of the budget of the National Resources Fund for specialized therapies)	

Intangible Cost

Intangible cost such as pain, anxiety, inconvenience and other factors which diminish QoL are equally enormous as direct and indirect cost, and are frequently unquantifiable. In several situations with chronic diseases, personal relationships, leisureliness and flexibility can also be negatively influenced. Treatment can be time-consuming, inconvenient and uncomfortable. Persons with chronic diseases may have difficulty in obtaining jobs, in the workplace, they can face discrimination, and professional life may be curtailed because of impediments of disease, such as early disability and death. However, data regarding the economic burden of intangible costs for chronic diseases are scarce.

The rising prevalence of chronic diseases continues to threaten the economies of developing countries. The economic burden of chronic diseases might actually be much worse in developing countries than developed countries, but the data are still scarce. Projections reveal that more than $7 trillion will be lost from the four major chronic diseases in low-middle-income countries (LMIC) between 2011 to 2025; averaging roughly US$500 billion (bn.) annually. The presence and growing prevalence of chronic diseases in developing countries will continue to present primary stumbling blocks to economic growth. Global estimates for CVD in 2010 were US$863 bn., which is projected to increase to US$1,044 bn. in 2030. The number is equally daunting for diabetes; the global cost was approximately US$500 bn. in 2010. Intangible cost such as pain, anxiety, inconvenience and other factors which diminish QoL are equally enormous as direct and indirect cost, and are frequently unquantifiable. In Burkina Faso, financial difficulties increased by 50% in households affected by chronic disease. The economic burden of chronic disease emphasizes the need for initiatives to prevent and control chronic disease prevalence and their devastating complications.

Part II: Healthcare System, Governments and Non-Healthcare Systems

Chapter 3

Can Healthcare Systems in Developing Countries Cope with Chronic Diseases?

Background

Health systems in developing countries continue to face considerable challenges in providing high-quality, affordable and universally accessible care (Lewis et al., 2012). The exponential growth of chronic disease in developing countries will place more stress on their existing fragile health care systems. For example, in South Africa, roughly 15% of the population have chronic kidney disease (CKD) and roughly 20,000 people needed treatment for kidney disease in 2012 (de Jagar 2012). Most of the developing countries are dealing with the double burden of communicable (infectious) and chronic diseases. Presently, developing countries must address the double burden (Bradshaw and Steyn, 2001). One of the challenges for developing countries is to reorient their healthcare systems toward managing chronic diseases. To effectively deal with chronic diseases, developing countries must adjust healthcare systems priorities to incorporate a chronic-disease prevention approach.

Health systems incorporate all the organizations, institutions and resources directed to producing health actions whose primary intent is to improve health. Primarily, health systems include: i) service provision. Service provision comprises of public or private formal and informal service providers, and also service organizations at the level of service delivery and higher up the chain of management (WHO, 2000); ii) resource generation, which includes human resources, physical capital, and drugs and medical supplies; iii) financing includes the volume and sources of financial resources available for the health system, and the procedures for pooling resources and transferring them to service providers; and iv) stewardship is the role of oversight of the health system, which falls to the government. It includes defining the vision and direction of health policy, exerting influence through regulation, and the collection and use of key data (WHO, 2000).

Curbing the chronic disease epidemic necessitates a multifaceted health systems response, which needs to be maintained across a gamut of care (Samb et al., 2010). WHO (2007) has defined health systems as all organizations, people, and actions with the primary purpose of promoting, restoring and maintaining health (Figure 17). The independent set of building blocks in Figure 17 interacts to accomplish the intermediate objectives, access coverage and efficiency, and the overall goals and outcomes. It should be noted that the building blocks are generic to all health systems (Figure 16). However, they do not serve as a one size fits all for the different countries; their organization in each country is dependent on cultural issues such as history, politics and social values (Duran et al., 2014). Furthermore, Samb et al. (2010) stated that an effective health system facilitates any individual, irrespective of: i) their place of residence; ii) their social and economic situation to access appropriate, high quality primary care services; and referral to secondary and tertiary care as necessary without the likelihood of financial hardship.

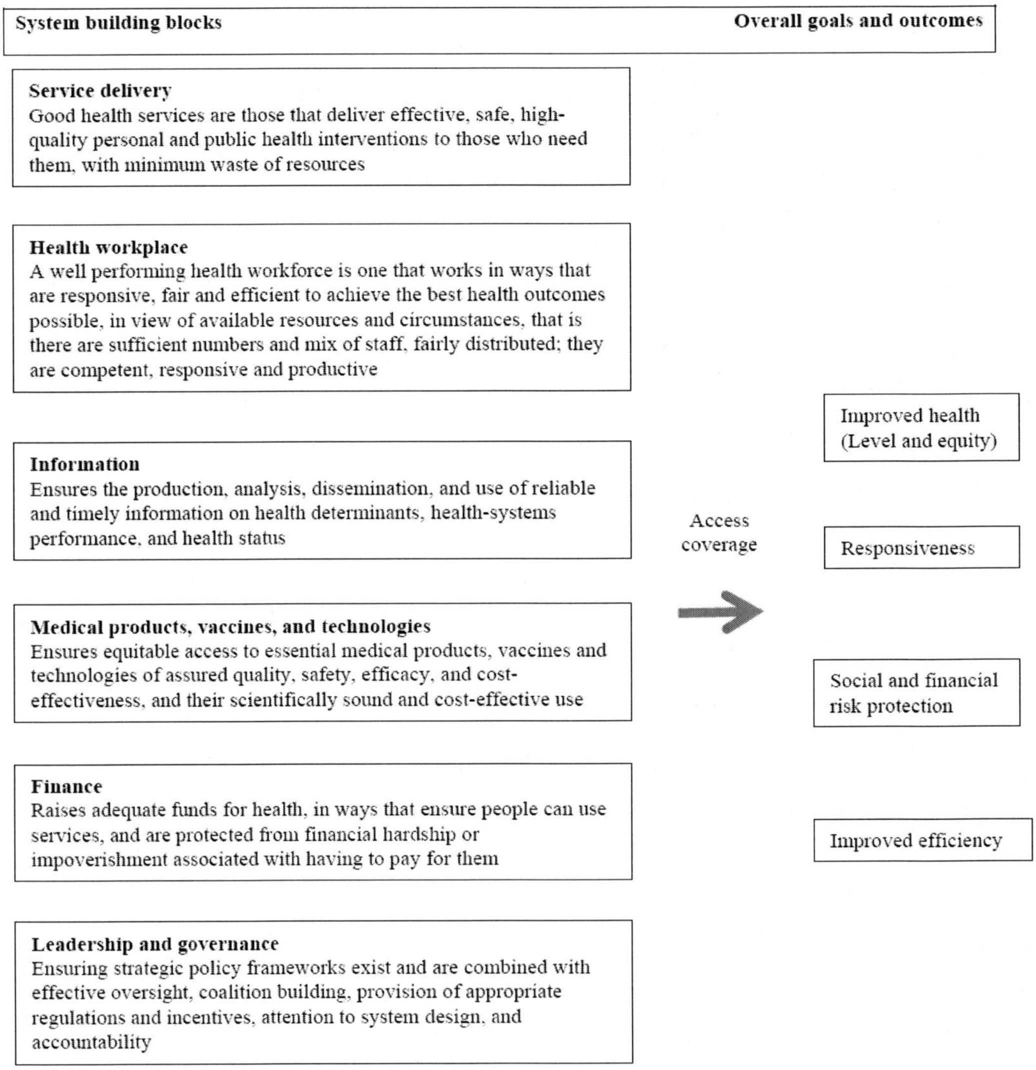

Figure 17. What is a health system? (Samb et al., 2010; Duran et al., 2014).

Largely, health services are categorized as: i) primary, secondary or tertiary health care, although some systems may also have additional levels of separation. Primary care is usually the first point of contact for a patient, where most preventative health can be achieved and early diagnosis can be possible (Starfield 2001). Primary care involves interactive communication with patients, community visits, outreach health promotion programs, and preventative strategies. Primary health care is usually a cost-effective strategy for decreasing escalating chronic disease, which demands long-term care and strong community support. For example, the WHO (2008) estimated that effective use of existing preventive measures could reduce the global burden of disease by as much as 70%. Table 10 summarizes some of the differences between primary and traditional health care model utilized by developing countries.

Table 10. Comparing conventional health care with people-centered primary care

Conventional ambulatory medical care in clinics or outpatient departments	Disease control programs	People-centered primary care
Focus on illness and cure	Focus on priority diseases	Focus on health needs
Relationship limited to the moment of consultation	Relationship limited to program implementation	Enduring personal relationship
Episodic curative care	Program-defined disease control interventions	Comprehensive, continuous and person-centered care
Responsibility limited to effective and safe advice to the patient at the moment of consultation	Responsibility for disease-control targets among the target population	Responsibility for the health of all in the community along the life cycle; responsibility for tackling determinants of ill-health
Users are consumers of the care they purchase	Population groups are targets of disease-control interventions	People are partners in managing their own health and that of their community

(WHO, World Health Report, 2008).

Challenges Facing Health Systems in Developing Countries

Health System Model

Traditional health care systems in developing countries are largely based on a model for treatment of acute illness (communicable or infectious disease); they are hospital-based. The orientation of health care systems to acute conditions results in fragmented care, erratic medication supplies, resource problems, and lack of sustainable services for chronic disease prevention and control. As shown in Table 11, this traditional health care model utilized by developing countries lacks appropriate health promotion initiatives, and disease prevention education services to effectively address the escalating chronic disease problem (Beaglehole et al., 2008; Bradshaw and Steyn, 2001). Comprehensive care of chronic diseases incorporates primary prevention, screening, secondary prevention, rehabilitation and palliative care with emphasis on mental health (WHO, 2013).

Table 11. Attributes of effective care for chronic conditions (PAHO, 2013)

OUTDATED CARE	EFFECTIVE CARE
Disease-centered	Disease-centered
Specialty care/hospital-based	Primary health care–based
Focus on individual patients	Focus on population needs
Reactive, symptom-driven	Proactive, planned
Treatment-focused	Prevention-focused

Lack of Appropriate Medicines

Developing countries rarely have the appropriate medicines necessary to treat chronic diseases. For example, dispensing long-term medications for chronic disease is seldom organized so that patients can obtain refills in an efficient manner (Bradshaw and Steyn, 2001). Mendis et al. (2007) examined the affordability and availability of medicines in six developing countries and reported that, in Malawi, the cost of one month of combination treatment for CHD was equivalent to 18·4 days' wages for the lowest-paid government worker. Higuchi (2009) and Beran et al. (2008) revealed that many patients diagnosed with diabetes faced multiple barriers to continued care in the Philippines and Viet Nam. Barriers such as the inability to undergo laboratory tests and the high cost of prescription medicine prevent patients from gaining access to routine care and ultimately adherence to care.

Health System Workforce

Most health systems in the developing world give priority to training and expertise in communicable disease (de-Graft Aikins et al., 2010; Flessa, 2003). Citing Africa as an example, there is generally a lack of adequately trained healthcare workforce in developing countries. On average in sub-Saharan Africa, there are 2.2 physicians per 10,000 people versus a ratio of 33.2 physicians per 10,000 persons in Europe (Morhason-Bello et al., 2013). Again, in sub-Saharan Africa, there are 9.0 nursing and midwifery personnel per 10,000 persons versus 65 per 10,000 population in Europe (Morhason-Bello et al., 2013). Shortages and deficiencies in education and training for the prevention, detection and treatment of chronic diseases prevent good outcomes. For example, a diverse workforce with highly specialized primary health care workers, tertiary-care professionals and public health specialists for screening, interventions, and identification of behavioral changes is often needed. Deficiencies in training allow for fragmented use or widespread failure to utilize guidelines. Poor patient–provider communication has also led to insufficient understanding of illness for both sides (Goudge et al., 2009). In the situation where there is lack of skilled health workers, those who are present are mostly concentrated in the urban areas. Also, poor retention rates due to the negligible salaries paid to the skilled health workers impact negatively on the health systems. Additionally, the working conditions are usually adverse for their health. As a result of the foregoing, there are limited numbers of health workers in developing countries with specialist training and knowledge in chronic diseases. Chronic disease reduction requires the development of new training formats.

Lack of Basic Medical Equipment, Diagnostic Tests

In developing countries hospitals and clinics frequently lack basic medical equipment for effective diagnosis and treatment of chronic diseases (de-Graft Aikins et al., 2010). Radiotherapy machines are the basic equipment necessary to provide radiation treatment in cancer (Abdel-Wahab et al., 2013). Researchers have established an association between the number of radiotherapy machines per million people and gross national income per head. The number of teletherapy machines per million people is an indicator for access to radiation therapy for a given region (Abdel-Wahab et al., 2013). In 2010, the average number of teletherapy machines per million people was: 1.99, 8.6 1.6, 0.71 and 0.21 for the world, high-income countries, upper-middle income countries, lower-middle income countries and low-income countries, respectively (Abdel-Wahab et al., 2013; Table 1). Roughly 10 developing countries and approximately 100 million people have been reported to have no radiotherapy unit to access to cancer treatment (WHO, 2010). Low budgetary allocations in health generally lead to low spending on medical equipment.

According to WHO (2010), in some countries, shortages of needles, syringes, and sterilizing equipment mean that up to 40% of injections are unsafe. Table 12 shows the availability of basic diagnostic (urine and blood) tests. Essential urine and blood tests were unavailable in primary care in some countries (Mendis et al., 2012). WHO (2010) has outlined other factors which further complicate the medical equipment problem such as: erratic power supplies, uncertain water quality, a shortage of health personnel, limited training capacity, difficulties in getting spare parts, and poor or inadequate maintenance. Another challenge in health systems is the lack of recognition of the new challenges of chronic diseases, and therefore the lack of medical equipment for patients' self-monitoring.

Table 12. Percentage availability of basic diagnostic tests in primary care facilities in defined areas in eight countries, 2009/2011 (Mendis et al., 2012)

Urine and blood tests	Benin (n = 12)	Eritrea (n = 6)	Sudan (n = 12)	Syria (n = 14)	Bhutan (n = 7)	Sri Lanka (n = 14)	Vietnam (n = 15)	Suriname (n = 10)
Urine albumin	100	67	92	64	100	46	0	70
Urine glucose	92	67	92	71	100	54	0	70
Urine ketones	42	33	58	79	0	0	0	40
Blood glucose	67	17	75	93	0	0	0	90
Blood cholesterol	25	0	33	14	0	8	0	20
Serum creatinine	33	0	58	0	0	8	0	10
Serum troponin	8	0	8	0	0	0	0	0

Limited Budgetary Allocations

In many developing countries, the health system is often inadequate due to insufficient allocation of resources by governments, and inadequate infrastructure creating lack of access and affordability of preventive care to the population (Ibrahim and Damasceno, 2012). Furthermore, in sub-Saharan African countries, roughly 80% of the inadequate healthcare budget is allocated to acute communicable diseases (Morhason-Bello et al., 2013). Healthcare budgets in developing countries face many challenges. For example, in sub-Saharan Africa, the total per head expenditure on all healthcare costs combined is less than US$100 per person versus US$7,000 - 9,000 per person in the U.S., Luxembourg and Switzerland (WHO, 2012a).

According to the Economic Intelligence Unit (2014), more than 30 sub-Saharan systems have annual per capita spending of less than US$100 on health, including both public and private money.

It should be noted that there is great variation in the percentage of governments' expenditure out of the GDP, allocated to health. To demonstrate: Bhutan allocates about 3.6% of its expenditure to health, countries in Africa5%; 10 - 12% in Asia; and 17.1% in the U.S. (World Bank, 2015).

Globally, annual government expenditure on health ranges from less than US$ 10 to over US$ 7,000 per person (WHO, 2010). The WHO reports that sub-Saharan Africa has 11% of the world's population and 25% of the global burden of disease, but accounts for less than 1% of global health expenditure. Contrastingly, the Americas have 14% of the worlds' population, 10% of the global burden of disease and more than 50% of the global health expenditure (INCTR, 2014).

In the 2014 global status report on non-communicable diseases, WHO (2014) revealed that 6% of countries had no funding for chronic disease activities. South Africa, the wealthiest of the sub-Saharan African (SSA) countries, has less than one doctor per 1,000 people. Uganda has one physician for every 8,547 people (WHO, 2012a). Only two countries of 52 in SSA have a substantial budget for chronic diseases. In general, insufficient budgetary allocation impacts on all areas of the healthcare system including equipment, personnel and distribution, which in turn negatively affects chronic disease prevention and management (Hanna 2008).

In most developing countries, public and private spending is inadequate to provide the quality health care needs of their populations. To illustrate, treatments, which are extremely cost-effective in developed countries, such as antihypertensive drugs, are unaffordable to most affected people in developing countries. Approximately 80% of diabetes care is provided in the developed countries versus 20% of diabetics who survive in developing countries (IDF, 2007).

Comprehensive care of chronic diseases incorporates primary prevention, screening, secondary prevention, rehabilitation and palliative care with emphasis on mental health (WHO, 2013). The implementation of effective, low-cost comprehensive programs to combat chronic diseases is dependent on availability of sufficient funds. Funds are required to sustain population-wide primary care interventions such as screening, and high cost interventions such as dialysis (Samb et al., 2010).

Workload and the Capacity of the Health System

Another factor influencing the quality of care for chronic conditions is the workload and the capacity of the health system to effectively meet the needs of those seeking care. Overcrowded waiting rooms and clinics may be commonplace in many settings because of the increased number of patients seeking care for chronic diseases. A rational use of the available resources for the management of CNCD is thus critical. For example an adequate amount of health provider's time is needed for medical encounters to effectively carry the myriad of tasks required for chronic care, including medical and psychological management, self-management support and data collection, among others (PAHO, 2013a).

Lack of Universal Health Care Coverage

The importance of universal health care (UHC) in chronic disease prevention cannot be overemphasized. Chronic diseases would best be dealt with by a universal, patient-focused health system based on primary care (The Economist Intelligence Unit, 2014). For example, in the last two decades, Rwanda, East Africa has slowly been building a UHC system with its 45,000 community health workers at the base. The rapidly improving health outcomes in Rwanda demonstrate the effectiveness of the UHC approach to communicable disease (The Economist Intelligence Unit, 2014).

UHC coverage in national health systems is central to effective prevention and control of chronic diseases (WHO, 2013). "The goal of universal health coverage is to ensure that all people obtain the health services they need – prevention, promotion, treatment, rehabilitation and palliation – without risk of financial ruin or impoverishment, now and in the future" (World Health Report, 2013). UHC offers an excellent opportunity to prioritize very cost-effective NCD interventions (WHO, 2014). However, the fragile health care systems in developing countries often do not meet the prerequisites for the implementation of UHC.

Some of the major barriers to UHC in developing countries include: i) the lack of resources (previously discussed); ii) overdependence on direct payments by people at the point of healthcare service. For instance, many households do not have the means to pay for any health care at all, especially for out-of-pocket costs at point of service. According to the World Health Report (2013), approximately 150 million people suffer financial calamity annually because of out-of-pocket payment for healthcare services. In developing countries, out-of-pocket payments account for 60% of health financing compared with only 20% in developed countries (Cisse et al., 2007). In Nigeria, almost two-thirds of patients failed to adhere to chemotherapy for cancer partly because of the cost of the drugs (Emoti and Enosolcase, 2008); and iii) inadequate, inefficient use and distribution of the available resources have also been cited as a barrier to UHC (WHO Report, 2010).

In the 2014 Global Status Report on non-communicable diseases, the WHO articulated the need for investment in health systems as an important element for improving chronic disease outcomes (WHO, 2014). The report pointed to several gaps in the health systems at the primary care level. Only few developing countries have implemented primary prevention programs, which would mitigate chronic diseases or delay their onset. Although, most developing countries continue to struggle with fragmentation and lack of UHC, some are taking a progressive approach with regard to healthcare reform.

The case of health-system reform in Mexico is highlighted to demonstrate the beneficial aspects of UHC. Mexico initiated healthcare reform in 2003 because of a number of problems, including: i) limited budgetary allocations to health by the government; ii) unfair allocation of public resources; and iii) poor equipment and infrastructure in the healthcare system (Frenk et al., 2006; Knaul et al., 2012; Knaul and Frenk, 2005). The reform aimed to achieve UHC coverage that included the uninsured population (Goss et al., 2013). Components of the Mexican healthcare reform include funding for community health services, and a national public health insurance program (Seguro Popular), which provides access to essential health services and specialized interventions (Goss et al., 2013).

Seguro Popular provides funding for certain types of cancers including breast, testicular and prostate cancer (Goss et al., 2013). The program currently covers 52.6 million Mexicans and is continuing to increase the number of diseases covered (Knaul et al., 2012). The health-system reform in Mexico has positively impacted on cervical cancer screening, which has increased from 30% coverage in 2000 to 48.5% in 2012 (Goss et al., 2013).

Primary Healthcare

The prevention, management and control of chronic diseases cannot be effectively addressed without a well-run, sustainable primary healthcare (PHC) approach. As a matter of fact, investment in all levels of care, that is, primary, secondary and tertiary is a major component of chronic disease program. The Alma Ata declaration defined PHC as: *"essential health care based on practical, scientifically sound and socially acceptable methods and technology made universally accessible to individuals and families in the community....It forms an integral part of the country's health system...and of the social and economic development of the community...bringing health care as close as possible to where people live and work, and constitutes the first element of a continuing health care process. It is the first level of contact of individuals, the family and the community with the national health system, bringing health care as close as possible to where people live and work, and constitutes the first element of a continuing health care service"* (www.who.int).

The Alma Ata declaration outlined eight elements, which are the underlying principles for comprehensive PHC program interventions to achieve the goal of health improvement (www.who.int). These elements include: i) education on prevailing health problems and methods of preventing and controlling them; ii) promotion of food supply and proper nutrition; iii) an adequate supply of safe water and basic sanitation; iv) maternal and child health care including family planning, immunization against major infectious diseases; v) appropriate treatment of common diseases and injuries; and vi) the provision of essential drugs. However, Dennill et al. (1998) indicated that if PHC is to be successfully implemented, it must take into consideration the tenets outlined below.

- **Political commitment**: The presence of progressive political will is central to the success of a health system.
- **Integration of** health promotion, curative, preventive and rehabilitative health care services.
- **Equity:** Everyone must have equal access to basic health care and social services without segregation of sub groups and provision of care.

- **Accessibility:** Services must reach all people in the country in terms of geographical, financial and functional accessibility.
- **Affordability:** Level of health care must be in line with what the community and country can manage to pay for. The inability to pay should not be a limiting factor to receiving health care.
- **Availability:** There should be adequate and appropriate services to meet particular health needs of each community.
- **Effectiveness:** Services provided must meet the objectives for which they were intended and should be justifiable in terms of cost.
- **Efficiency:** Results accomplished should be proportionate to resources used (www.who.int).

Since the Alma Ata declaration, some countries, such as Brazil and Cuba have successfully implemented the PHC approach to deliver health services, while others as Zambia and South Africa continue to encounter challenges, which hamper their progress. Older studies from Black (1990) and Dennill et al. (1998) have stressed that most successful comprehensive PHC programs demonstrate good government policies and legislature for equitable implementation of efficient and cost-effective health care interventions with the inclusion of community and individual participation. According to the WHO, Brazil is a case in point.

Brazil's health care system is based on decentralized universal access, with local Governments providing comprehensive and free health care to each individual in need. This is financed by states and Federal Government. One aim of the federal, state and municipal governments in Brazil is to encourage underserved citizens to utilize and benefit from the PHC system through the Family Health Program; the country's main PHC strategy. PHC is one of the main pillars of the public health system in Brazil; about 70% of its population receives care from this system.

Cuba is another example of a country taking a progressive approach. Cuba's PHC is unique because it is law (policy), and it is the vehicle through which all health systems are run. Community initiatives drive the Cuban PHC system; the communities are involved in the diagnosis of their health problems and identify their health priorities. In collaboration with Government representatives, individuals develop strategies and action plans to address the community health diagnosis priorities (Magnussen et al., 2004).

In an effort to improve health outcomes following the Alma Ata Declaration, most developing countries established PHC implementation strategies. However, several challenges have impeded the execution of these PHC strategies in developing countries. Examples of these impediments include: declining GDP, inadequate health budgets, lack of political will, and increased burden on health care services (Ohoimbo 2003). The case of Zambia, taken from (Magawa 2012) is used to demonstrate the challenges faced by developing countries in their efforts to implement PHC.

"In Zambia, PHC implementation began in August 1981, with steady progress and interventions that included the training of community health workers, construction and upgrading of rural health centers, improved distribution of medicine, a strengthened transport system, as well as improved health planning and management. These interventions were largely driven by the economic boost that Zambia experienced due to the increase in the global demand for copper - Zambia's main export product and the country's major source of income at the time. This progress was, however, short lived. When global demand for copper fell significantly, it had a severely negative effect on the country's GDP. The health sector experienced a shortage of health staff and deteriorating health services and infrastructure. In addition, there was little or no action by the Government to redistribute the available resources more equitably to districts with the greatest health need - especially in rural areas. Even basic health promotion and prevention activities, which had shown to be effective, such as health education, could not be sustained."

The lack of political will is another major deterrent to successful implementation of the PHC approach in developing countries. "For example, South Africa was a worldwide leader in the conceptualization and development of the PHC concept. However, despite going through years of structural reform and sincere commitment to achieving health for all, the slow response by Government to provide equitable and quality health services to all individuals has hampered progress in achieving the desired health outcomes. This was aggravated by the intimidating state interventions during the apartheid era and weak leadership in the health sector post-independence, particularly related to the decentralization of health services, poor infrastructure and services, and inequities in resource allocation and distribution. As a result, the country is faced with a quadruple burden of disease, that is, increased cases of non-communicable diseases tuberculosis, high maternal and child death and others" (Magawa, 2012; Kautzky and Tollman, 2009). More recently the South African Government has introduced a National Health Insurance (NHI). The aim of NHI is to promote universal access to appropriate, efficient and quality health services. The NHI has comprehensive PHC as one of its key features. A key approach of the NHI is to ensure that health care is available to everyone as geographically close to them as possible (NHI, 2011).

In sum, effective, sustainable PHC implementation, which is an integral part of any successful health system, requires the following major components: i) cost-effective measures; ii) equity; iii) community participation; and iv) political commitment (Magawa, 2012). Once these components are in place, PHC appears to be a good strategy to achieve health for all.

Improving the Efficiency of Healthcare Systems

Developing countries need to get really creative if they are to provide good quality chronic disease care, given the predicament of their healthcare systems. These countries will need to adapt models for chronic care, make them country-specific and select particular features for implementation. The WHO Strategy for chronic disease prevention suggests that a stepwise approach can be positively affected.

Various models for chronic disease management have been suggested for countries with inadequate resources to carry out all the recommended actions. One of Davey et al.'s (2015) suggested approach is the progressive integration of care for chronic conditions into primary care activities. However, in doing so the capabilities of the healthcare system must be taken into consideration. Such approaches will probably: i) give better outcomes in attempts to improve chronic disease care; ii) help to address problems such as resource constraints; and iii) identify and allow for capitalization and implementation of certain attributes of the people, the health system and the country. Generally, if these approaches are well applied, increasing numbers of people with chronic disease have been propositioned and executed globally.

Three chronic care models are described. Over a decade ago, the Chronic Care Model (CCM) was proposed by Wagner et al. (1999) and Wagner et al. (2001) to prevent complications and improve management and outcomes in patients with chronic diseases. The underlying principle of CCM is the restructuring of medical care through partnerships between health systems and communities, and the empowerment of patients with self-management skills and tracking systems. As shown in Figure 18, the CCM encompasses six areas for improvement and provides a structure for organization/practice change. In totality, these CCM areas are meant to create more effective health care delivery systems, with solid foundations for decision support, linkage of health care systems to community resources and policies, delivery of comprehensive self-management support services for patients, and operation and management of patient-centered clinical information systems.

Research has indicated that the implementation of the CCM in developed countries verified significant correlations between certain elements of the CCM and better health outcomes (Coleman et al., 2009; Nutting et al., 2007). Additionally, a number of studies have shown that when care is consistent with the elements of the CCM quality of life and outcomes for patients with diabetes are better (Nutting et al., 2007; Parchman et al., 2007a; Schmittdiel et al., 2008; Kirsh et al., 2007; Parchman et al., 2007b; Williams et al., 2010). However, the number of elements of the CCM and the type and intensity of implementation may vary, depending on circumstantial and administrative factors (Cretin et al., 2004).

The Innovative Care for Chronic Conditions (ICCC) Framework is an expanded version of the CCM produced by the World Health Organization in 2002 (Figure 19). The ICCC gives greater emphasis to community and policy aspects of improving health care for chronic disease (WHO, 2002b; Epping-Jordan et al., 2004).

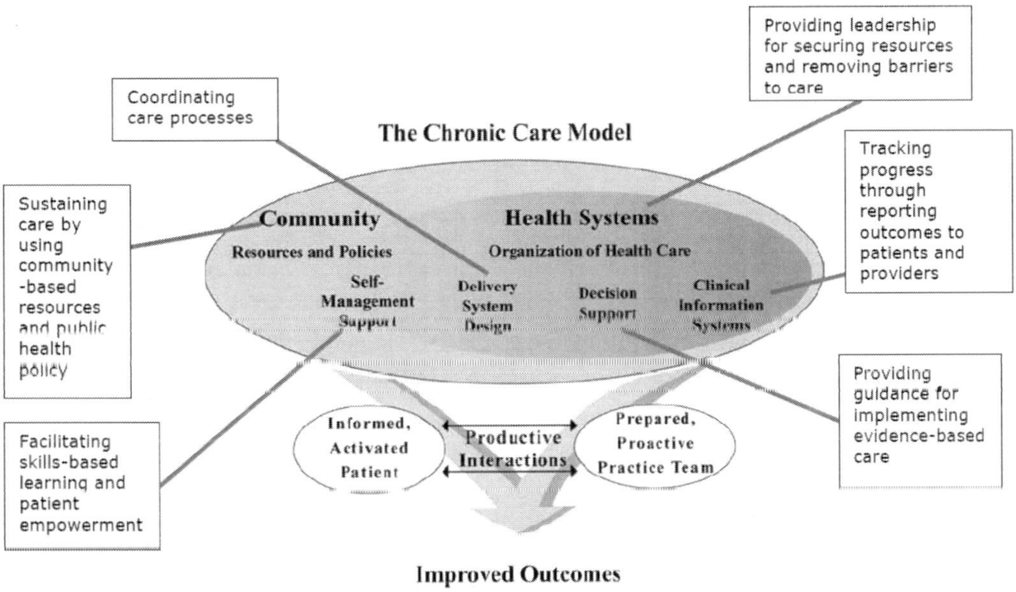

Figure 18. The Chronic Care Model (modified from Bodenheimer et al., 2002).

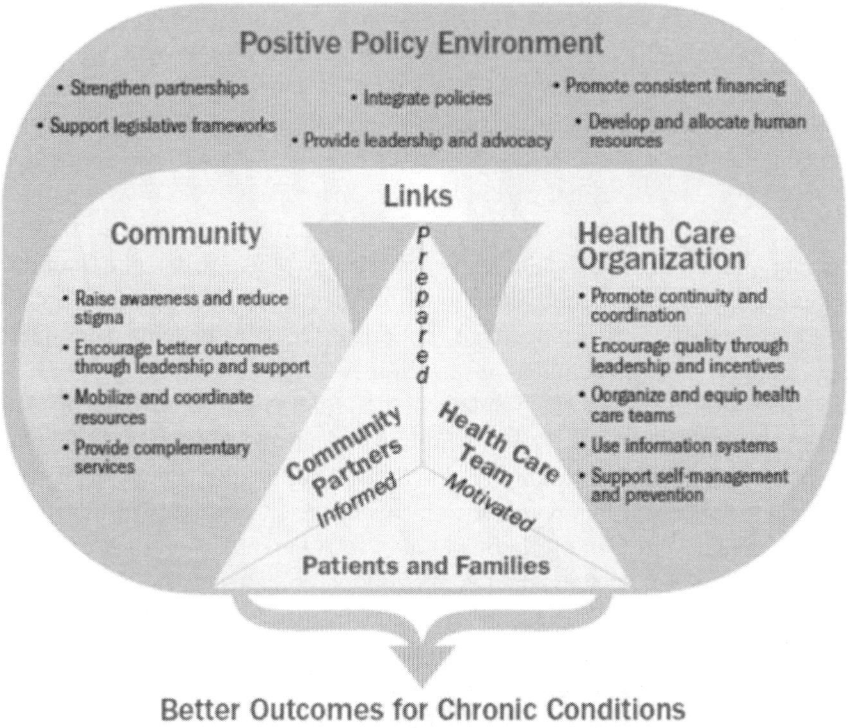

Figure 19. Innovate Care for Chronic Conditions Framework (PAHO, 2013a).

The Expanded Chronic Care Model (ECCM) extends the role of healthcare systems and providers outside clinical settings. Most behaviors, which impact health, occur in individuals' communities. It is therefore critical to recognize how social determinants of health affect adherence to preventive therapies in chronic disease prevention (Ockene et al., 2011). The ECCM has three additional components relevant to the community: i) building public health policy; ii) creating supportive environments; and iii) strengthening community action (Figure 20).

Ockene et al. (2011) suggested four approaches, which could be incorporated into the ECCM to improve the use of preventive therapies for cardiovascular health: i) improve access; ii) increase implementation and translation; iii) provide links between clinical and community-based therapies; and iv) increase patient demand and utilization (Figure 21). These are also applicable to other chronic diseases. The approaches are discussed in detail in Ockene et al. (2011).

Curbing the chronic disease epidemic necessitates a multifaceted health systems response, which needs to be maintained across a gamut of care. Health systems in developing countries continue to face considerable challenges in providing high-quality, affordable and universally accessible care. The WHO estimated that effective use of existing preventive measures could reduce the global burden of disease by as much as 70%. In developing countries, the orientation of health care systems to acute conditions results in fragmented care, erratic medication supplies, resource problems, and lack of sustainable services for chronic disease prevention and control. Some of the challenges facing healthcare systems in developing countries include: the health system model used, lack of appropriate medicines, basic medical equipment and diagnostic test, weak health system workforce, limited budgetary allocations, poorly run or no PHC and the lack of UHC. Barriers such as the inability to undergo laboratory tests and the high cost of prescription medicine prevent patients from gaining access to routine care and ultimately adherence to care. There are limited numbers of health workers in developing countries with specialist training and knowledge in chronic diseases.

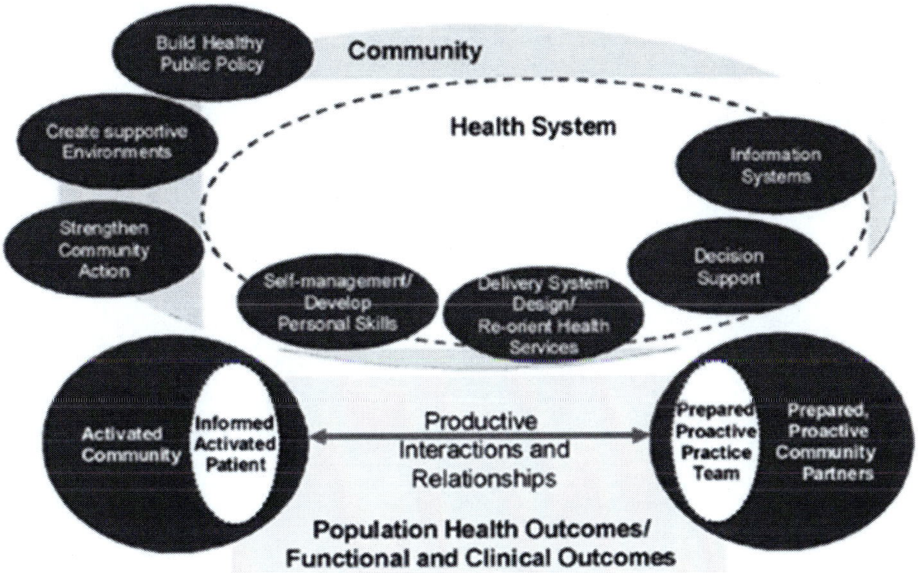

Figure 20. The Expanded Chronic Care Model (Barr et al., 2011).

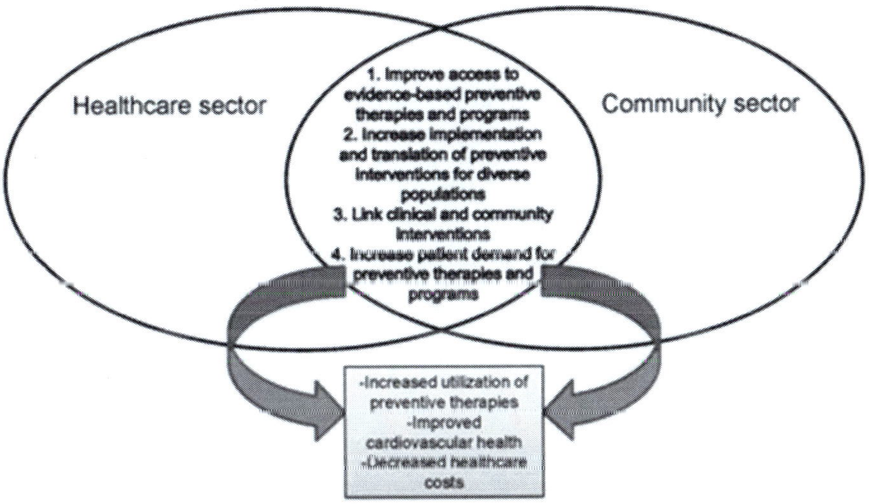

Figure 21. Strategies to improve use of preventive therapies for cardiovascular health (Ockene et al., 2011).

Roughly 10 developing countries and approximately 100 million people have been reported to have no radiotherapy unit to access cancer treatment. In sub-Saharan African countries, roughly 80% of the inadequate healthcare budget is allocated to acute communicable diseases. Various models for chronic disease management have been propositioned and executed globally. Research has indicated that the implementation of the CCM in developed countries verified significant correlations between certain elements of the CCM and better health outcomes. The ICCC gives greater emphasis to community and policy aspects of improving health care for chronic disease. The ECCM extends the role of healthcare systems and providers outside clinical settings. Developing countries must begin to select the model(s) most appropriate to their situation and begin to implement aspects of these models if they are to curb the rising chronic disease problem, which is threatening their sustainable development.

Chapter 4

Governments and Chronic Disease

Current State of Affairs

The discussion is taken from: "Financing national NCD responses in the post-2015 era Preliminary recommendations from the WHO Working Group on Financing for NCDs" (Interim Report released on the occasion of the Third UN Conference on Financing for Development [Addis Ababa, 13-16 July 2015]; available at: http://www.who.int/global-coordination-mechanism/wg_financing_interimreport)

Governments should play leadership role in the prevention, management and control of chronic diseases. Five years ago (2011), Heads of State and Government acknowledged that chronic diseases is one of the major public health problem in the world. In 2015, world leaders adopted the Sustainable Development Goals (SDGs), which include targets to, by 2030, reduce by 33% premature mortality from chronic diseases through prevention and treatment (Appendix A). The number of countries which had operational chronic disease policy with the appropriate budget for implementation jumped from 32% in 2010 to 50% in 2013.

However, these countries indicated that commitments were often not translated into action in developing countries owing to a lack of national capacity. To counteract this problem, the WHO Working Group on Financing for NCDs recommends a considerable increase in chronic disease financing over the next 15 years. This would include financing for technical assistance and capacity building to developing countries, through domestic, bilateral, regional and multilateral channels, including traditional and voluntary innovative financing mechanisms. WHO is insisting that Heads of State and Government must honor their commitments made in 2011 to explore the provision of adequate, predictable and sustained resources.

At the Third UN International Conference on Financing for Development (Addis Ababa, 13-16 July 2015) for NCDs in the post-2015 era, some preliminary recommendations and suggested actions with their supporting arguments were made. The recommendations, facts and supporting arguments clearly highlight the problems; demonstrate government's position in most developing countries, and their commitment to chronic disease prevention and control. The recommendations are summarized below.

Recommendation 1: Significant additional investments are required to attain the NCD-related targets included in the SDGs by 2030.

Facts and supporting arguments

- The total cost for implementing a set of very cost-effective and affordable NCD interventions in all developing countries would be US$ 11 billion annually.
- A recent WHO and World Bank Group report revealed that 400 million people do not have access to essential health services and 6% of people in developing countries are tipped into or pushed further into extreme poverty (US$1.25/day) because of out-of-pocket payments for health services.
- Inadequate public funding for health services make out-of-pocket payments the single largest component of domestic funding in many developing countries, accounting for 48% and 36% of total health expenditure in low- and middle-income countries, respectively in 2012. The negative impact of out-of-pocket payments on families has been discussed earlier in this book. From 1995 to 2013, government spending on health increased from 3.4 to 4.1% of GDP on average across 190 countries. The increase in low-income countries has been faster, from 1.7 to 2.6% of GDP. The challenge now is to help low- and lower middle-income countries find ways to mobilize and increase the effective use of domestic public resources for health funding.
- WHO estimates that to scale up priority health services towards UHC would need a minimum additional spending of US$55 billion by 2030 in 34 low- and 48 lower middle-income countries.

Recommendation 2: These additional investments to implement national NCD responses will need to rely primarily on domestic public resources.

Facts and supporting arguments

- Public spending on health can increase in two ways, either: i) government overall raises more tax revenues; or ii) government devotes a greater share of its available funds to health
- Raising tobacco taxes will generate extra public revenues, reduce consumption, improve health, slow the grow of health care costs, protect poor people, and combat poverty
- Specific high-priority, very cost-effective and affordable interventions are already well described in the WHO Global NCD Action Plan 2013-2020

Recommendation 3: Equally important, these additional investments for NCDs require scaled up and more effective Official Development Assistance (ODA) to complement efforts of countries to mobilize resources domestically.

NCDs continue to receive the smallest amount of ODA funding for all major global health areas, accounting for 1.2% of health development assistance for health 20. International development cooperation will need to financially support domestic efforts in the poorest countries to achieve the NCD-related targets included in the SDGs by 2030.

Facts and supporting arguments

- WHO's global country capacity survey (CCS) on the prevention and control of NCDs conducted in 2000, 2005, 2010 and 2013 confirm that low-income countries lack the capacity to generate or leverage domestic resources such as taxes on tobacco and alcoholic beverages
- Expressed as a proportion of current health care spending, the average annual cost of implementing a set of very cost-effective and affordable NCD interventions amounts to 4% in low-income countries (compared to 2% in lower middle-income countries and less than 1% in upper middle-income countries)
- The Addis Ababa Accord provides important messages on scaling up and more effective international public finance to complement the efforts of countries to mobilize resources domestically from other sources, public and private, including from improved tax collection.

Recommendation 4: Promoting investment from private business and finance in areas critical to addressing NCDs is also important, including contributions from philanthropists.

Facts and supporting arguments

- Heads of State and Government committed themselves in 2011 to call upon the private sector to (i) reduce the impact of marketing of unhealthy foods and non-alcoholic beverages to children, (ii) produce and promote more products consistent with a healthy diet, (iii) create an enabling environment of healthy behaviors among workers at the workplace, (iv) reduce the use of salt in the food industry, and improve access to and affordability of NCD medicines and technologies To date, progress in fulfilling this commitment has been largely absent
- WTO/TRIPS allows WTO Members to protect public health and improve access to affordable essential medicines for developing countries, but it is not clear that these approaches are being pursued in any systematic way
- The Addis Ababa Accord provides important messages on the importance of investment from domestic and international private business and finance in areas critical to sustainable development, including contributions from philanthropists.

Recommendation 5: There are also opportunities to resolve the coherence and consistency of financial, investment, trade, development and public health policy.

Facts and supporting arguments

- The Addis Ababa Accord is concerned about policy incoherence and agrees to resolve the coherence and consistency of multilateral financial, investment, trade, and development policy and environment, institutions and platforms, and increase cooperation between major international institutions, while respecting mandates and governance structures

- Preliminary investigation by the Working Group has revealed that a number of global health initiatives are engaged in innovative support for NCD prevention and treatment. However, these innovations are happening due to the entrepreneurial efforts of country-based staff from WHO and other UN agencies, the World Bank or international NGOs. These organizations work with Ministry of Health officials in the various countries to find solutions, rather than using a systematic approach to health system strengthening, delivering on UHC targets, or responding to the growing burden of NCDs. Improved policy coherence and alignment would support universally agreed aid effectiveness principles and facilitate achievement of NCD targets with relatively little additional investments.

How Governments Can Take the Lead

If governments in developing countries are to be effective in reducing the burden of NCDs and meet their targets agreed upon through the World Health Assembly, then they need to take action similar to those suggested for obesity by the International Obesity Task Force. IASO (2014) describes how government can take the lead by building the case for intervention; encouraging advocacy and developing social marketing campaigns; and making interventions to reduce poor dietary intake and protect consumer health. The list of suggested interventions for governments is summarized.

Strengthen the case for action (IASO, 2014)

- Monitor and predict national productivity losses and health costs, accumulated throughout the life cycle from the burden of chronic diseases, and assess the economic case for taking action.
- Monitor progress and change in relation to the drivers of chronic diseases.

Develop cross-departmental action plans embracing a broad range of initiatives at multiple levels of intervention (IASO, 2014)

- Establish inter-departmental taskforces to coordinate government strategies to tackle chronic diseases, considering all aspects of food supplies and nutrition security, the physical environment and secure physical activity.
- Review relevant policies and evidence for their effectiveness and cost-effectiveness.
- Review policy success and failures in related areas of public health promotion and protection, and interventions to achieve behavior change.
- Involve public health and civil society organizations in developing strategies and action plans, and providing evidence of good practices.
- Develop a systems-based analysis of opportunities for intervention at multiple levels.

Establish guidelines and standards for prevention of chronic disease (IASO, 2014)

- Monitor and strengthen standards for commercial practices which threaten nutrition and physical activity security.
- Monitor and strengthen standards for the provision of food in state-controlled institutions.
- Support the construction of operational tools including nutrient profiling schemes, food formulation standards, food environment indicators, health impact assessments.

Use government purchasing power to build healthier consumption patterns (IASO, 2014)

- Support the inclusion of health and nutrition criteria for awarding government supply contracts.
- Use school and hospital food policies as beacons of good practice in the community.

Use government legislative powers to strengthen public health legislation (IASO, 2014)

- Review and strengthen public health legislation in order to allow increased intervention across market sectors for public protection.

Use multilateral negotiation opportunities to strengthen national health programs (IASO, 2014)

- Negotiate better health protection through cross-border agreements on marketing.

Encourage behavior change and a shift in cultural norms (IASO, 2014)

- Use social marketing to encourage changes in cultural norms and to build public acceptability for interventions.
- Disseminate examples of good practice from other countries.

Strengthen Ministry of Health leadership (IASO, 2014)

- Ministries of Health need to demonstrate a strong business case for public health action, especially fiscal action such as taxes and subsidies to influence purchasing patterns, and market interventions on advertising, prices and labeling.
- Ministries can demonstrate their obligations to follow international charters and agreements (for example, for tobacco) and recommendations from authorities such as WHO.

Gather support and counter resistance (IASO, 2014)

- Ministries can demonstrate popular support from non-governmental organizations, including health and consumer advocacy groups but also pro-family and child interest groups (e.g., churches, charities) and campaigns by parents/mothers networks.

- Ministries can counter resistance from commercial interests by making more transparent the role and activities of commercial lobbyists and political donors.

Establish accountability agencies (IASO, 2014)

- Establish independent agencies which can monitor and report publicly on policy development, implementation and progress towards targets.
- Extend accountability for health impact to other sectors, including the commercial operators and their federal bodies, non-governmental organizations and the media.

Individual Countries/Governments/Regions Efforts to Prevent Chronic Diseases

Kenya - UN, Kenyan government take broad-based approach to fighting NCDs (Available at: http://www.who.int/nmh/events/2014/kenya-ncd-prevention)

Chronic diseases account for 27% of deaths suffered by Kenyans aged between 30 and 70 years, equivalent to almost 370,000 people annually. This reduces productivity, curtails economic growth and traps the poorest of poor in chronic poverty. The probability of dying too young from a chronic disease in Kenya is 18%. The main risk factors for chronic disease in Kenya are the same as elsewhere in the developing world, that is, harmful use of tobacco and alcohol, physical inactivity and unhealthy diets, due to effects of globalization on marketing and trade, rapid urbanization and population aging. Chronic diseases contribute to over 50% of inpatient admissions and 40% of hospital deaths, which dominate health care budgets in Kenya.

The UNIATF was established by the UN Secretary-General in 2013 and placed under WHO's leadership. It is coordinating the activities of the relevant UN organizations and other intergovernmental bodies to help realize the 2011 Heads of State commitments in the 2011 Political Declaration on chronic diseases, in particular by implementing the WHO Global Action Plan for the Prevention and Control of Non-communicable Diseases 2013–2020. The responsibility for tackling chronic diseases lies with government, but action requires extensive collaboration across government and with a broad range of development partners.

The Kenyan government and the UN Country Team are collaborating to address the country's rising number of premature deaths from chronic diseases, including heart diseases, cancers, diabetes, and chronic respiratory diseases, scaling up solutions based on national leadership, global perspectives and local insights. The government and the UN Country Team received support from the United Nations Interagency Task Force for the Prevention and Control of chronic diseases (UNIATF) to help build and share solutions in three main areas:

- Setting national targets for chronic diseases.
- Finalizing the work on the development of a national action plan to reduce exposure of Kenyans to risk factors for chronic disease thus enabling health systems in Kenya to respond to chronic disease.
- Mapping the chronic disease epidemic to ensure that they are no longer hidden, misunderstood and underreported.
- The aim is to reduce the vast number of premature deaths for chronic disease in Kenya in line with WHO voluntary global target of a 25% reduction in premature mortality from chronic diseases by 2025.

The UN Country Team and the Joint Task Force on chronic diseases are trying to scale up programming for chronic diseases. This will lay some groundwork for policy development and strategies required develop appropriate programs to address chronic diseases s prevention and management. The Kenyan government has prioritized chronic disease prevention and control in the following: i) National Medium Term Plan (MTPII) 2014-2018; ii) National Health Strategic Plan (KNSSP) 2014-2018; iii) the just-launched United Nations Development Assisted Framework (UNDAF) 2014-2018 for Kenya; and iv) the Kenya third generation WHO Country Cooperation Strategy (2014-2019).

The Joint Mission of the UNIATF has encouraged Kenya to make prevention the cornerstone of the national response to chronic diseases. The Task Force met with senior Kenya health officials responsible for chronic diseases, health promotion, community health and tobacco control. The Task Force also met with representatives of academia and civil society, officials from Kenya's ministries of Labor and Social Security; the Treasury, Information, Communication and Technology; Transport and Industrialization; Land Housing and Urban Development; and Education; plus the Tobacco Control Board and National Authority for the Campaign Against Drug and Alcohol Abuse.

Strong partnerships across multiple ministries of government, and between governments, communities and the private sector, are essential. Prevention must be the cornerstone of any national response to chronic diseases. A set of cost-effective interventions to prevent and control of chronic diseases exist in all countries. Some studies estimate that implementing these very cost-effective interventions will cost only 4% of current health spending in low-income countries, 2% in lower-middle-income countries and less than 1% in upper-middle-income countries.

Caribbean: Declaration of Port-of-Spain: Uniting to stop the epidemic of chronic NCDs (Samuel et al., 2014)

The Caribbean Community (CARICOM) is composed of 15 member states and five associate members. CARICOM members have a combined population of 17 million and an average life expectancy ranging from 70 to 80 years except in Haiti, where it is 62 years (Caribbean Community Secretariat, 2013). The Caribbean region has the highest burden of chronic diseases in the Americas (Caribbean Community Secretariat, 2013). In 1986, the Caribbean Cooperation in Health Initiative, approved by health ministers made chronic diseases a priority concern (Hospedales et al., 2011). The CARICOM heads of government identified chronic disease among other things as regional priorities in the 2001 Nassau Declaration. At this time they called for strategies for the prevention and treatment of NCDs and outlined principles and processes to preserve and enhance "the health of the Region which is the wealth of the Region" (Caribbean Community Secretariat, 2011). In 2005, the Caribbean Commission on Health and Development reported that the number of deaths from diabetes, hypertension and heart disease combined was 10 times higher than the number of deaths from acquired immunodeficiency syndrome (AIDS) and declared NCDs a "super priority" (Caribbean Community Secretariat, 2006a).

At the 2006 CARICOM Summit, governments received a report on the macro-economic implications of non-communicable diseases" and agreed to host a special regional consultation on compliance with specific recommendations pertaining to tobacco, diet and physical activity (Caribbean Community Secretariat, 2006b). In 2007, CARICOM heads of government participated in the CARICOM Summit on Chronic Non-Communicable Diseases, which was held in Port of Spain, Trinidad and Tobago. Eleven heads of government and five ministers present agreed that "immediate collective actions were necessary to manage and control chronic diseases and a 15-point summit declaration titled *Uniting to stop the epidemic of chronic NCDs* (also known as the Declaration of Port of Spain) was issued (Caribbean Community Secretariat, 2007). The declaration called for policies and actions for the prevention and control of the four major chronic diseases and their common risk factors (Appendix B). Regional and multilateral organizations and the independent, authoritative scientific and academic community were represented at the CARICOM Summit, but there was inadequate representation of NGOs. Funding for follow-up actions was insubstantial (Samuel et al., 2014).

In 2009, chronic diseases were on the agenda of the Fifth Summit of the Americas. Leaders agreed that they could reduce the burden of chronic diseases through: i) the promotion of comprehensive and integrated preventive and control strategies at the individual, family, community, national and regional levels and ii) through collaborative programs, partnerships and policies supported by governments, the private sector, the media, civil society organizations, communities and relevant regional and international partners. A grid for the reporting of countries' compliance with the 15 mandates of the Declaration of Port of Spain was revised in 2010 (Appendix C).

The 2011 compliance (using the reporting grid, Appendix C) reports were mixed with a mean score of 53%. The countries with the highest implementation scores were, in order, Barbados - 82%, Trinidad and Tobago - 72%, Bermuda - 71.5% and Dominica - 69%. The countries with scores below average were Saint Vincent and the Grenadines - 27.5%, Anguilla - 19.5% and Haiti - 8.5% (Samuel et al., 2014).

Factors, which could reduce compliance, include natural disasters, for example, the 2010 earthquake in Haiti (Samuel et al., 2014) diverted the country's attention towards the immediate crisis. The global economic crisis that started in 2008 created barriers to compliance (Samuel et al., 2014). The trend in the CARICOM Summit is that countries with a higher GNIs and GDPs and larger populations are more likely to follow through on their commitments than those with lower GNIs and GDPs or smaller populations (Samuel et al., 2014). Commitments supported regionally, such as Caribbean Wellness Day, or internationally, such as commitments related to the FCTC, are also more likely to be fulfilled (Caribbean Community Secretariat, 2011). Samuel et al. (2014) concluded that an accountability mechanism based on annual reporting is critical for monitoring progress and highlighting areas in need of correction.

The Political Aspect of Chronic Disease

Stuckler and Siegel (2012) write extensively about the politics of chronic diseases. Readers are referred to this extensive document. Some of the key points of their discussion are highlighted here.

Lack of funds and resources available for chronic disease control (Stuckler and Siegel, 2012)

- Less than 3% of $22 billion in global health funds went to chronic diseases in 2007.
- WHO, allocates about 9% of its budget to NCDs.
- Roughly 50% of all global health money comes from private foundations or companies.
- Monies are routed through budgeting systems, which are often inconsistent and difficult to track Close to 33% of the money earmarked for health is spent on unidentifiable activities.
- The misalignment between health needs and health allocations is the greatest for private donors, who assign the least priority to chronic diseases. Many of these private donors have potential conflicts of interests, as they are in close contact with, sit on the boards of, or own substantial shares in food and pharmaceutical companies.
- Ultimately, the failure to prioritize and act on chronic diseases is more of political than technical.

Governments must take the lead in the fight against chronic diseases, building the case for intervention; encouraging advocacy and developing social marketing campaigns; and making interventions to reduce poor dietary intake and protect consumer health. The literature provides a vast majority of suggested interventions, which governments, if they have the political will could adopt to meet their country's needs.

Chapter 5

Non-Health Systems: Interactions and Partnerships for Chronic Disease Prevention

Generally, the professional healthcare system in the developing world is faced with many challenges. The developed countries have provided evidence of effectiveness that incorporation of the concepts of health promotion, self-care and community participation in healthcare systems lead to improvement in the health status of populations (Bhuyan 2004).

Community participation (CP) emphasizes the "bottom up" approach in planning and implementation of development programs including health development, where people are seen as active participants, compared to the conventional "top down" approach, where people are considered as passive recipients of programs designed for them by professionals and Government officials (Oakley 1989). The underlying themes of both these issues are the involvement and empowerment of people in promoting and caring for their own health. Plumb et al. (2012) noted that the potential to significantly improve prevention and decrease morbidity and mortality from chronic diseases could be enhanced by effectively engaging communities using established principles of community engagement.

Rationale for Community Partnerships in Chronic Disease Management

Chronic diseases are multifaceted in that they have physiological, sociocultural and political standpoints (Plumb et al., 2012). It is a momentous task to manage chronic conditions through a cycle of fragmented measures, such as physician office visits, public health announcements, government funded programs, individual service programs or the establishment of community advocacy groups (Plumb et al., 2012). In order to ascertain the underlying causes of the many facets, which put individuals at risk for chronic diseases, an all-inclusive approach is required. This all-inclusive approach should involve community engagement for problem definition and partnership development to characterize and instigate efficient, sustainable solutions and management policies (Plumb et al., 2012).

Social Ecology Theory and Community Partnerships

The Social Ecology Model (SEM) of health promotion provides an important framework for integrating community partnerships and chronic disease management (Stokols, 1996). The theory indicates that the potential to change individual risk behavior is considered within the social and cultural context in which it occurs (Goodman et al., 1996). The SEM recognizes the multifaceted interaction among individual, relationship, community, and societal factors. The overlapping rings in the model shows how factors at one level impact those at another level (Box 1). Additionally, the SEM reveals that in order to bring about positive health change these interrelations must be recognized and addressed. The model also suggests that in order to prevent chronic diseases, it is necessary to act across multiple levels of the model at the same time. This approach is more likely to sustain prevention efforts over time than any single intervention (CDC, 2015).

Box 1. Social Ecology Model (CDC, 2015)

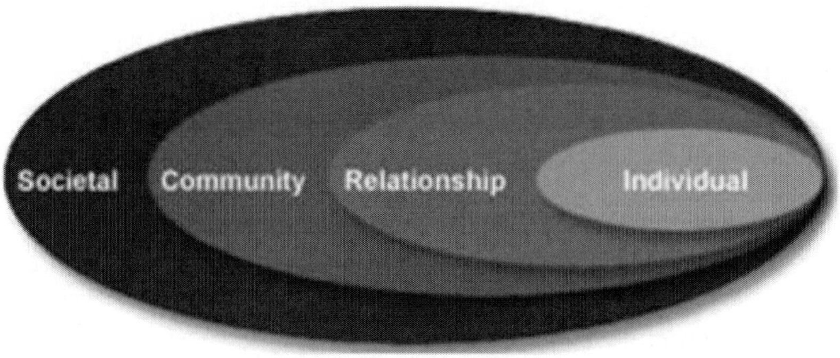

Chronic diseases usually share the same underlying root cause of disease for example, physical inactivity and inadequate diets. The following example of the SEM demonstrates a project "Building Community Support for Diabetes Care (BCS) of the Robert Wood Johnson Foundation (Brownson et al., 2007). The BCS required that projects build community supports for diabetes care through clinic-community partnerships, by addressing four key areas: 1) working with existing services, encouraging use of these services and enhancing access to them; 2) working together to identify gaps and create new programs, services, or policies that complement existing services; 3) providing leadership and a forum to raise awareness about diabetes and create consumer demand for resources and supports; and 4) providing a forum for community input and participation (Brownson et al., 2007). Examples of BCS interventions by ecological level are shown in Box 2. Brownson and colleagues (2007) concluded that BCS projects using partnership approaches show promise for building community support for diabetes care. Other chronic diseases will benefit from continued support for implementation and evaluation of partnerships to build community supports for self-management. Plumb et al. (2012) have detailed multiple examples of local and national case community-based partnerships.

Box 2. Ecological Level BCS Interventions (Plump et al., 2012)

Individual:	Diabetes education classes, supermarket tours, case management, community walking maps, cooking demonstrations
Family, friends and peers	Family diabetes curriculum, support groups, peer led education classes
Systems/organizations	Office staff training to enhance capacity to support diabetes self-management, physician prescription pads for referrals to walking clubs, creation of health care performance goals
Community/Policy	Advocacy training for project workers, securing indoor spaces for physical activity, diabetes materials in public libraries, presentations to community organizations to increase awareness of diabetes, improved selection of fresh produce at local markets

To curb the global increase in chronic diseases, a social ecology approach should be implemented. This calls for the promotion of new linkages between the traditional medical system and issues such as economic development and access to healthy and affordable food. 26, Providers can become directly involved in providing technical expertise and/or advocating in a variety of ways for changes in social policies that effect health (Gruen et al., 2006; Woolf, 2000). The ECCM in Figure 20 provides the groundwork to investigate these extended roles and operationalize the social ecology approach. Many evidence-based examples in improving chronic disease management and outcomes in diabetes, obesity and hypertension have been shown in the literature (Lee et al., 2008).

Interacting with Private Sector and NGOs to Reduce Chronic Diseases

Although governments and countries need to lead the effort to prevent, treat, and manage chronic diseases, this epidemic requires a coordinated response from multilateral organizations, civil society, and the private sector. The knowledge of multinational companies and leading NGOs could be garnered to assist with the chronic disease reduction. Such action has the potential to enable families to find healthier food options and enable more health workers to provide quality services to people in rural areas. Sturchio (2014) has articulated five ways that the private sector and their partners can and are working to reduce the burden of chronic diseases. Three of these are repeated as examples of the collaboration in this book:

- **Strengthening the health workforce**. An estimated 1 billion people have never seen a health worker. The private sector is bringing its expertise in attracting and retaining talent to bear by supporting governments and NGOs in helping to strengthen human resources for health. One example is the Clinton Global Initiative's (CGI) partnership between Medtronic, one of the largest medical device companies, and the NGO Last

Mile Health to support the integration of chronic disease training and diagnosis in Liberia (Sturchio 2014).

- **Creating healthier product offerings.** Working in collaboration with civil society, governments, and multilateral agencies, companies can move toward making healthier products more readily available. In Latin America, for example, a number of countries have effectively partnered with the food and beverage industry to reduce the salt content in bread (Sturchio 2014).
- **Building healthy cities.** Economic development and urbanization go hand in hand to create a subsequent rise in chronic disease rates. Cities and governments can invite various commercial entities to help reduce indoor and outdoor pollution, build healthier buildings, and create pedestrian-friendly streets (Sturchio 2014).

Abbato (2008) examined the potential role of NGOs in the prevention, detection and management of chronic disease on the Gold Coast with a focus on the four chronic disease targeted for initial action by the Queensland Strategy for Chronic Disease (T2D, CVD, renal disease and CRD). The following five key strategies provide a summary of the findings:

- **Establish NGO alliances related to chronic disease**

Build strong collaboration across NGOs to share information, improve marketing and communication, increase coordination, reduce fragmentation and competition and implement collaborative projects.

- **Streamline referral pathways**

Improve information provided by physicians and at hospital discharge, implement approaches such as chronic disease practice nurse model to facilitate timely access to needed services and supports

- **Provide assistance for social connections and depression**

Increase understanding, awareness and support in acknowledgement of the critical role they play in achieving positive prevention and self-management of chronic disease

- **Increase the focus on prevention, screening, risk factor management, early intervention**

Work together to find ways to increase the level of activity and investment within existing resources and activities and influencing policy and funding priorities

- **Partner to fill identified gaps**

Work with groups and agencies which have much to offer in respect of current gaps in support and services in respect of chronic disease.

Abbato (2008) outlined several recommendations regarding NGOs ranging from data collection, social support and networks, detection and screening initiatives, programs and services for chronic disease management, and health promotion collaboration including government initiatives. Examples of the role of NGOs in chronic disease prevention and control are shown below.

Example 1: The Public Health Responsibility Deal (England) (IASO Policy Briefing, 2014)

An example of a voluntary public-private partnership is the Department of Health England's 'Public Health Responsibility Deal' which coordinates a series of voluntary industry commitments and pledges on food, alcohol, physical activity and healthy workplaces, including civil society organizations. The government considered this approach would be faster and cheaper than regulation, and some progress has been made, for instance with the introduction of smaller portion size options for soft drinks and confectionery. Experience with public-private partnerships suggest that such schemes need strong monitoring and evaluation with clearly agreed definitions and areas of action, independent standards-setting with sanctions or targets (Petticrew et al., 2013; Panjwani and Caraher, 2013). Civil society organizations have been cautious to offer support to the Responsibility Deal, especially around proposals regarding alcohol consumption, with most preferring to call for regulatory measures (Triggle, 2011; Limb, 2013).

Example 2: Bloomberg Uses Philanthropic Support to Promote Change through Community Action (IASO Policy Briefing, 2014)

Bloomberg Philanthropies has launched an Obesity Prevention Program to support community advocacy and popular awareness-raising (Bloomberg Philanthropies, 2013). The Foundation's $10m support for obesity prevention in Mexico is designed to promote what the organization believed are the policies likely to have the most impact:

- Banning junk food and sugary beverage advertising to children
- Raising taxes on sugar-sweetened beverages
- Promoting healthy public sector food policies
- Introducing front-of-package nutrition labels
- Developing obesity prevention advertising campaigns

The 3-year program includes subway advertising campaigns in Mexico City depicting the negative effects of obesity, TV ads calling for a tax on soft drinks, media stories in popular newspapers and in social media, and research reports on children's exposure to commercials, the foods and beverages available in schools, and the national economic damage caused by obesity. Within the first year of the Bloomberg supported program, the Mexican government had introduced an 8% tax on 'junk' food and a 1 peso tax per liter of soft drinks (Anon 2013).

Part III: Chronic Risk Prevention – Manipulating Common Modifiable Risk Factors

Chapter 6

Diet, Nutrition, Physical Activity and Chronic Diseases

The risk factors for chronic diseases have been discussed earlier in this book. This chapter takes a more in-depth look into two of the most common, modifiable risk factors, namely, unhealthy diets and physical inactivity (Table 5). These risk factors are lifestyle related and can be prevented. Figure 22 shows the microsimulation model (chronic disease prevention [CDP] model) developed by the OECD and WHO (Sassi et al., 2009). The model implements a so-called causal web of lifestyle risk factors for selected chronic diseases (Sassi et al., 2009). As shown in Figure 22, the risk factors go from more distal to proximate exposures, which are more immediately connected to disease events. It also shows the major relations between risk factors and chronic diseases and the shared interactions between risk factors. The proximal risk factors directly affect the probability of developing the mentioned chronic diseases, while the distal risk factors intermediated in part by body mass index (BMI) have an indirect impact on chronic diseases.

Tobacco and alcohol abuse and control have been discussed in detail elsewhere (Gaziano and Pagidipati, 2013; John, 2008). The phenomenon of nutrition transition has also been discussed earlier in this book. It has been shown that globally, people are consuming more energy-dense foods, which are rich sources of saturated fats, trans fats, sugars, and salt. Concomitantly, as people change their eating habits, they are consuming less fruits, vegetables and dietary fiber, which are key components of a healthy diet. It has been well established that adoption of a healthy diet, adequate physical activity and smoking cessation could reduce up to 80, 90 and 33% of cases of CHD, type 2 diabetes and some types of cancers, respectively (Hooper et al., 2012).

Basic Principles of a Healthy Diet

A healthy diet helps protect against chronic diseases and malnutrition in all its forms (WHO, 2015). Constituents of a healthy diet includes: i) balanced energy intake and expenditure to prevent unhealthy weight gain (Hooper et al., 2012; FAO, 2010); ii) consumption of free sugars should be limited to less than 10% of total energy intake (WHO,

2015). WHO (2015) recommends a further reduction to less than 5% of total energy intake for additional health benefits; iii) salt intake less than five grams per day helps prevent hypertension and reduces the risk of heart disease and stroke in the adults (WHO, 2014); and iv) less than 30% of total energy intake from fats (Nishida 2009). Unsaturated fats, such as those found in fish, avocado, nuts, sunflower, canola and olive oils are preferable to saturated fats found in butter, cream, cheese, ghee and lard (Nishida 2009). Optimally, intake of saturated fatty acids should be limited to <7 - 10% of total calories (Nishida 2009). Trans fatty acids consumption should be maintained at <1% of total calories, and dietary cholesterol to <200 mg/day (IAS, 2015). High intakes of industrial trans fats such as those found in processed, fast and fried foods, frozen pizza, pies, cookies, margarines and spreads are inconsistent with a healthy diet (Nishida 2009). This book will emphasize the relationship between chronic disease and selected dietary constituents (salt, sugars and cholesterol).

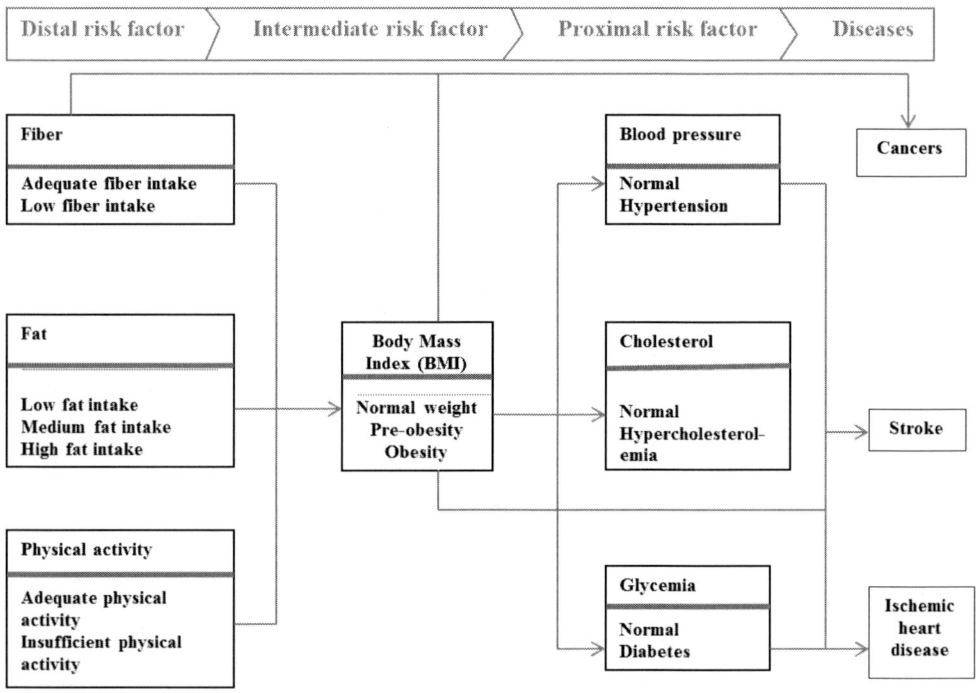

Figure 22. Causal web for risk factors and disease events implemented in the chronic disease prevention model (Cecchini et al., 2010; Sassi et al., 2009).

Dietary Factors Which Affect Chronic Diseases

Sodium Intake and Cardiovascular Disease

An unhealthy diet is one of the major risk factors for some of the most common chronic diseases, such as CVD, cancer, diabetes and other conditions linked to obesity.

Sodium is an important mineral and electrolyte, with many biological functions including transmitting nerve impulses, contracting and relaxing muscle fibers, and maintaining proper fluid balance in the human body.

In conjunction with potassium, sodium also plays a crucial role in blood pressure regulation. It is estimated that for essential physiological functions, adolescents and adults need a minimum daily intake of 500 and 850 mg sodium and chloride, respectively, which corresponds to 1.3 g of salt per day (Bochud et al., 2012).

A high consumption of sodium has been repeatedly linked with hypertension, which is a risk factor for CVD (He and MacGregor, 2013; Graudal et al., 2011; Figure 22). Table 13 shows the global cardiovascular deaths attributed to sodium consumption >2 g/d in 2010, by gender, country income, and selected world regions. Additionally, high sodium consumption (>2,000 mg/day, equivalent to 5 g salt/day) in combination with insufficient potassium intake (<3.5 g/day) also contribute to hypertension, heart disease (HD) and stroke. Salt is the primary source of sodium in our diet.

However, sodium can come from sodium glutamate a flavor enhancer, used in foods in some parts of the world, and other food additives such as sodium benzoate. Health Canada (2012) reported that 88% of all the sodium in Canadians' diets come from food manufacturing or preparation and is not present naturally.

Mozaffarian et al. (2014) estimated that in 2010, the average global sodium intake was 3.95 g/person/per day. Overall, in 181 of 187 countries, adults consumed >2,000 mg or 2 g salt/day. WHO's recommended limit for daily sodium intake is <2,000 mg/day for adults (Mozaffarian et al., 2014).

Figure 23 shows the average sodium intakes (g/day) in 2010 in 21 Global Burden of Diseases regions. It has also been reported that in 2010, four of every five sodium-associated deaths from CVD causes occurred in low-income and middle-income countries. Globally, 17.8% of the premature deaths from CVD causes were credited to sodium intake above the reference level.

In general, there are limited data regarding salt consumption across individual countries of Africa and other developing countries. However, in South Africa and Nigeria, daily salt intake averages roughly eight grams per day, which is well above the WHO's recommended limit of five grams/day (UK Department for International Development, 2011).

Reducing sodium intake

Reducing salt intake has been identified as one of the most cost-effective measures countries can take to improve population health outcomes (Bibbins-Domingo et al., 2010). WHO member States have agreed to reduce the global population's intake of salt by 30%, and halt the rise in diabetes and obesity in adults and adolescents as well as in childhood overweight by 2025 (WHO, 2012b; 2013; 2014). It is estimated that 2.5 million deaths could be prevented annually if global salt consumption were reduced to the recommended level.

Table 13. Global cardiovascular deaths attributed to sodium consumption >2 g/d in 2010, by sex, age, country income, and world region (Mozaffarian et al., 2014)

	Adults in millions	Average sodium g/day	Deaths per million adults per year attributed to sodium consumption >2 g/day				Percent of total CVD deaths per year attributed to sodium consumption >2 g/day			
			CHD	Stroke	Other CHD,	All CVD	CHD	Stroke	Other CHD	All CVD*
World	3,830	4.0	461	338	168	966	10.2	12.7	8.6	9.5
Women	1,930	3.8	321	259	140	720	8.7	10.7	7.3	8.0
Men	1890	4.1	600	417	196	1213	11.7	14.7	9.9	10.9
High-income countries	763	3.9	173	49	10	34	7.3	7.4	7.4	7.3
Upper-middle income countries	1,530	3.6	204	133	12	55	11.5	14.1	13.5	12.9
Lower-middle income countries	1,210	3.4	182	70	9	39	10.1	11.0	11.1	10.6
Low-income countries	323	2.9	77	56	7	24	8.7	9.5	8.8	9.1
Sub-Saharan Africa	320	2.5	130	221	102	453	6.6	8.2	5.4	6.0
Canada and the U.S.	226	3.6	337	92	108	537	8.6	10.7	7.2	8.0

*The numbers of deaths for each subtype may not exactly sum to the total CVD deaths due to rounding †In 2010 globally, there were 14,669,000 total CVD deaths, 6,963,000 CHD deaths, 5,798,000 stroke deaths, and 1,909,000 other CVD deaths. Among these events, values are the percentage of these deaths attributed to sodium consumption above the reference level. Income categorizations are based on the World Bank classification system (Table 1).

Sub-Saharan Africa: Angola, Burundi, Benin, Burkina Faso, Botswana, Central African Republic, Côte d'Ivoire, Cameroon, Democratic Republic of the Congo, Congo, Comoros, Cape Verde, Djibouti, Eritrea, Ethiopia, Gabon, Ghana, Guinea, Gambia, Guinea-Bissau, Equatorial Guinea, Kenya, Liberia, Lesotho, Madagascar, Mali, Mozambique, Mauritania, Mauritius, Malawi, Namibia, Niger, Nigeria, Rwanda, Sudan, Senegal, Sierra Leone, Somalia, São Tomé and Príncipe, Swaziland, Seychelles, Chad, Togo, United Republic of Tanzania, Uganda, South Africa, Zambia, Zimbabwe.

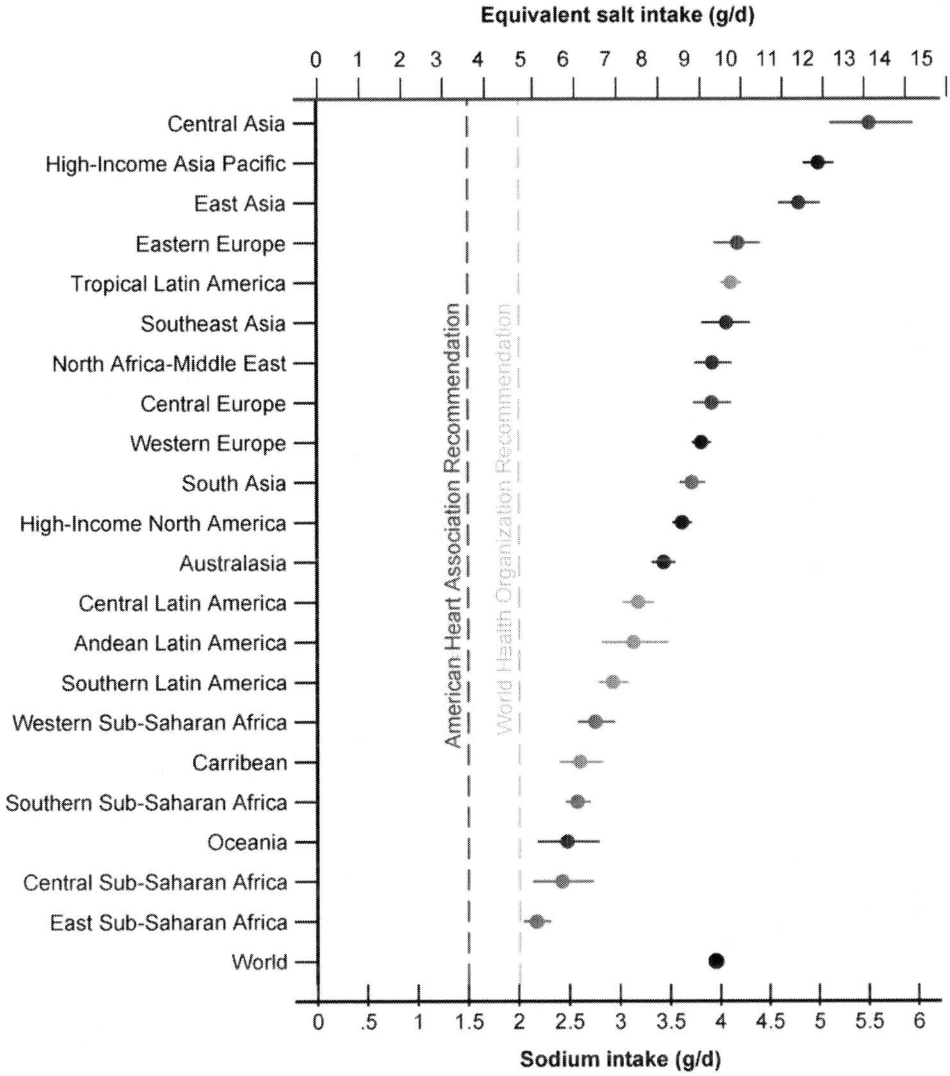

Figure 23. Mean (95% uncertainty interval) sodium intakes (g/day) in 2010 in 21 global burden of diseases regions (Powles et al., 2013).

Global Sodium Reduction Efforts

The principal benefit of lowering salt intake is a corresponding reduction in high blood pressure. Mozaffarian et al. (2014) have reported that each reduction of 2.30 g sodium per day was associated with a reduction of 3.82 mm Hg in blood pressure. Mandatory legislation restricting the salt content of selected foods have been proposed and implemented in some countries. This approach has been suggested to be 10 to 20 times more cost-effective than voluntary reductions in the U.S. and in Australian modeling studies (Cobiac et al., 2010; Bibbins-Domingo, 2010). Canada's food industry has been proactive in initiating sodium reduction in processed and packaged food products available for sale in the country. In addition, the Bureau of Nutritional Science, Food Directorate, Health Products and Food

Branch has provided further direction to the food industry to continue sodium reduction efforts and help Canadians achieve the average sodium intake goal of 2300 mg per day by 2016 (Health Canada, 2012).

Over time, some countries and regions have initiated various salt reduction strategies in an effort to lower the high incidence of CVD. In Finland, the food industry reduced the salt content of food products by 20 to 25%. This resulted in a 33% reduction in mean sodium intake; from 5,000 mg/day in 1980 to 3,300 mg/day in 2002. In turn, the reduced intake showed decreased systolic blood pressure by more than 10 mm Hg and 75% decrease in stroke and coronary heart disease mortality (Reinivuo et al., 2006; Karppanen and Mervaala, 2006). Between 1979 and 2007 a 36% decrease in salt intake was reported in Finland.

In the United Kingdom, the average daily intake of sodium decreased from 3800 mg in 2001 to 3440 mg in 2008 (Food Standards Agency, 2009). The European Commission's goal in 2008 was a 16% salt reduction over four years for all food products including salt consumed in restaurants and catering. Twelve categories of foods were identified as a priority; each member state chose at least five (European Commission, 2009).

More recent data revealed a 15% reduction in population salt intake and a decrease of 3/1.4 mm Hg in average blood pressure (Saddler et al., 2011; He et al., 2014). The New York City Health Department in collaboration with other stakeholders and food industry leaders initiated a voluntary nationwide effort in 2008 to lower the sodium content in processed and restaurant foods by 25%. They also aimed to for a 20% reduction in sodium intake in five years (New York City Department of Health, 2010).

Table 14. Types of salt reduction initiatives adopted by countries and regions (Trieu et al., 2015)

World Health Region	Number of countries
Africa	1
Americas	12
Eastern Mediterranean	2
Europe	34
South East Asia	5
Western Pacific	21
Type of salt reduction strategies used in the countries • Food reformulation mainly bread, bakery products, dairy products, processed meats etc. • Consumer education – raising awareness • Front of package labeling (FoPL) – logos and symbols for example, percent daily intake (%DI). Roughly 23 of the countries utilized this strategy. • Interventions in public settings (such as schools, hospitals, work place etc.) • Legislative initiatives such as taxing high sodium products – 25% of the countries employ legislative strategies.	

Trieu et al. (2015) identified 75 countries with national salt reduction strategies in 2014. Of these countries, 41, 21, 11 and one were high-, upper-middle, lower-middle and low-income, respectively (Table 14). The major strategies utilized included consumer education, food industry and front of package labeling (FoPL). The majority of the strategies are linked to chronic disease or nutrition programs (Trieu et al., 2015). The available data indicate that almost 66% of the European Region and 10 and 2% of the Eastern Mediterranean and African Region, respectively, have salt reduction initiatives. Furthermore, in South East Asia region, there are no voluntary or mandatory salt level targets to encourage reformulation (Trieu et al., 2015).

New York City to Require Salt Warnings on Menus

New York City's Board of Health has voted unanimously to require chain restaurants to put salt shaker symbols on menus to denote dishes with more than the recommended daily limit of 2,300 mg of sodium. New York is the first U.S. city with such a requirement. City officials indicated that consumers should know which menu items are high in sodium. The measure will apply to an estimated 10% of menu items at the New York city outlets with at least 15 outlets nationwide. The policy will go into effect on December 1, 2015.

Chilean Government-Led Voluntary Program for Food Reformulation

In 2011, the Chilean government and bakers agreed on a voluntary target for salt content in bread of 600 mg/100 g (IFPRI, 2015).

South Africa's Mandatory Limits on Salt Levels in Select Foods

In 2013, South African Department of Health adopted mandatory targets for salt reduction in 13 food categories (rolling implementation required by 2016 – 2019) (IFPRI, 2015).

Some potential salt reduction strategies to utilize in the home, communities and restaurants are shown below.

- No added salt during the preparation of food
- No salt shaker on the table; remove soy sauce and salt shaker from tables in restaurants
- Limiting the intake of salty snacks
- Selecting products with lower sodium content
- Integrating salt reduction into the training curriculum of food handlers
- Introducing product or shelf labels making it clear that certain products are high in sodium
- Providing targeted dietary advice to people visiting health facilities
- Advocating for people to limit their intake of products high in salt and advocating that they reduce the amount of salt used for cooking.

Although it has been well established that moderate reductions in sodium intake reduce the risk of high blood pressure, very few developing countries have initiated national salt reduction strategies in response to WHO's call for a 30% relative reduction in mean population intake of salt/sodium by 2025 in member states (WHO, 2013). Some of the successful salt intake reduction initiatives implemented in developing countries are reprinted in Table 15. The global action plan for the prevention and control of NCDs 2013-2020 suggested policy options for salt reduction, which include: i) implementation of WHO's recommendations on the marketing of foods; and ii) involvement of food industry to reduce the level of sodium added to prepared or processed foods (WHO, 2013). Only 2% of the African region and none in South East Asia region have initiated national salt reduction strategies.

Indeed, multisectoral collaboration is required to improve access to products with lower sodium content and ministries of Health in these countries need to take the lead. Health systems in developing countries should examine and adopt the suggested mechanisms to achieve sustained reductions in sodium intake at the population level in order to decrease chronic disease risk. The reduction of sodium intake is closely linked to WHO's global target of a 25% relative reduction in premature mortality from CVD, diabetes and CRD by 2025 – one cannot be accomplished without the other.

Sugar Intake and Diabetes

The global per capita sugar consumption has more than doubled over the past five decades (IDF, 2015). Over the last 10 years, global sugar consumption has grown from 130 to 178 million tonnes (WCRF, 2015). Roughly 75% of annual global sugar consumption takes place in developing countries (WCRFI, 2015). Sugar is found in virtually all processed foods, especially in sugar-sweetened beverages (SSBs). Several researchers have reported a strong linkage between high intake of SSBs (including fruit juice) and increased risk of type 2 diabetes (Barrio-Lopez et al., 2013; Koning et al., 2011; Malik et al., 2010). Utilizing a meta-analysis Wang et al. (2015) estimated that the risk of diabetes associated with high consumption of SSBs is 1.30 times more than that for low consumption. Evidence from The European Prospective Investigation into Cancer-InterAct study, which included eight European countries, revealed that one 12 oz. (354.9 mL) sugar-sweetened soft drink daily was associated with a risk of developing type 2 diabetes (InterAct consortium, 2013). It has also been reported that SSBs increase the risk of gestational diabetes (GDM) by 22% (Chen et al., 2009). In more than 50,000 women followed for eight years, those consuming more than one SSB per day had an 83% greater risk of developing T2D compared to those consuming less than one SSB daily (Schulze et al., 2004).

In the Nurses' Health Studies I and II, women who consumed four SSBs daily had a 44 and 28% higher risk of hypertension, respectively, compared with infrequent consumers (Winkelmayer et al., 2005). The Framingham Offspring Study found that individuals who drank more than one soft drink per day had a 22% higher incidence of hypertension compared with those who did not consume (Dhingra et al., 2007).

Table 15. National efforts to reduce population salt consumption are underway in many countries

Salt-Smart America (PAHO, 2013b)	National campaign to reduce salt consumption in Thailand In 2011 (Pattaya Mail, 2012)	Working with the private sector to reduce salt consumption in Argentina and South Africa (Ministerio de Salud Argentina, 2012)	Salt-reduction campaigns in Bahrain, Kuwait and Qatar (Kuwait News Agency, 2014)
The Pan American Health Organization (PAHO) initiative "Cardiovascular disease prevention through population-wide dietary salt reduction" supports countries of the Americas in reducing sodium intake, by providing effective tools, strategies and interventions. These include evaluating population-based salt intake, raising awareness, promoting voluntary salt reduction regulating salt use in manufacturing, improving food labeling, and promoting food science and health research. Since 2011, public health authorities in Argentina, Brazil and Chile in the south, and Canada, Mexico and the USA in the north have promoted voluntary national reformulation targets and timelines with the food industry. Most of these countries are targeting salt reduction in packaged foods and bread, while Mexico has focused on foods available in the school environment. Argentina has already achieved a 25% reduction in the salt content of bread. Keys to successful outcomes include voluntary salt reduction, education, health promotion, food labeling, regulation, ongoing monitoring, evaluation and reporting, research, and collaboration with the private sector.	The Ministry of Public Health of Thailand, along with other stakeholders, initiated a campaign aimed at reducing salt consumption by 50%. Academics and food producers jointly collaborate to undertake salt-reduction activities. Attention is mainly on foods for children, especially snacks. The academic sector collaborated with the commercial sector to reformulate snack recipes. However, the reformulated products were not acceptable to the public and gradually disappeared from the market. Consequently, a more successful approach was initiated, whereby food producers were asked to reformulate their products themselves. This strategy resulted in many good market products, such as potato chips with sodium reduced by 50%, and instant noodles with sodium reduced by 20% (using potassium chloride). When instant noodles with reduced sodium become widely available, this should have a significant impact, since this product is consumed widely – >8 million packages/day are sold to people of all socioeconomic classes.	The majority of WHO Member States have opted for setting voluntary targets for salt reformulation. However, others, including Argentina and South Africa, have opted for legislative regulation to set specific targets for various food groups. Both methods of adopting targets involve dialogue with the private sector to facilitate reformulation, and also require consumer awareness to enable informed consumers to make the full use of the enabling environment	The ministry of health of Kuwait established a national salt-reduction program in January 2013. The Salt and Fat Intake Reduction task force developed and implemented a national strategy to reduce salt consumption, in consultation with nutrition experts and scientists and officials from Kuwait's Food Standards Office, and in collaboration with the food industry. By the end of 2013, one of the food companies had reduced the salt content of bread – including white pitta bread, burger buns and whole-wheat toast – by 20%. Kuwait is exploring ways of reducing the salt content of another commonly consumed food item – cheese. The Qatar government is working with one of the country's major bakeries to reduce the use of salt by 20%, and Bahrain is setting up a similar campaign.

Daily soft drink consumers in the Framingham Offspring Study were found to have a 22% higher incidence of hypertriglyceridemia and low high-density lipoprotein (LDL) cholesterol compared with those who did not consume (Dhingra et al., 2007). Findings from the Multi-Ethnic Study of Atherosclerosis (MESA) study showed a significant effect of SSBs on hypertriglyceridemia, and trends toward an effect on hypertension and LDL cholesterol in daily SSB consumers versus those who did not consume (Nettleton et al., 2009). Also, cross-sectional analysis of National Health and Nutrition Examination Survey (NHANES) data found a positive association between SSB intake and blood pressure in adolescents (Nguyen et al., 2009). The Nurses' Health Study followed 88,000 women for 24 years and reported that those who consumed two SSBs per day had a 35% greater risk of developing CHD compared with those who consumed 1 SSB per month (Fung et al., 2009).

Additionally, Weeratunga et al. (2014) analyzed data from 165 countries and observed a strong positive correlation coefficient (0.599; $p < 0.001$) between prevalence of diabetes mellitus and per capita sugar consumption in all countries. Basu et al., (2013) have reported that per capita sugar consumption is directly and independently correlated to the occurrence of diabetes. Basu et al. (2013) found that every 150 kcal/person/day increase in sugar intake was associated with increased diabetes prevalence by 1.1% ($p < 0.001$). Fagherazzi et al. (2013) likewise stated that SSBs and artificially sweetened- beverages (ASBs) were associated with increased risk of type 2 diabetes. In developing countries, increased access to sugar may be partly responsible for the linkage observed between urbanization and increased risk of type 2 diabetes (Basu et al., 2013b; Cheema et al., 2014).

Singh et al. (2015) used comparative risk assessment methods and data on SSB intake from the Global Burden of Diseases multi-year study. Their estimates indicated that globally 184,000 deaths were attributable to SSB consumption, including 133,000, 45,000 and 6,450 due to diabetes, CVD, and cancers, respectively. Five, 70.9 and 24.1% of SSB-related deaths occurred in low-income, middle-income, and high-income countries, respectively (Singh et al., 2015). The authors concluded that SSBs are a major cause of preventable deaths due to chronic diseases in high-income and developing countries.

High Sugar Food, Sugar-Sweetened Beverages, Free Sugars

High sugar foods contain more than 22.5 g sugar per 100 g (xxxx17), based on total sugars within the product. It reflects the total amount of sugars in the product and also takes into account naturally-occurring sugars. Sugar-sweetened beverages are those that contain caloric sweeteners and include those listed in Table 16. Free sugars are include monosaccharides and disaccharides added to foods and beverages by the manufacturer, cook or consumer, as well as sugars naturally present in honey, syrups, fruit juices and fruit juice concentrates (WHO, 2015). The intake of free sugars should be reduced throughout the life cycle (WHO, 2015). Evidence indicates that in both adults and children, the consumption of free sugars should be reduced to less than 10% of total energy intake (WHO, 2015). Furthermore, WHO has indicated that a reduction of free sugars to less than 5% of total energy intake provides additional health benefits.

Table 16. List and definition of sugar-sweetened beverages (CDC, 2010)

Sugar-Sweetened Beverage (SSB)	Definition
Soft drinks or Soda, pop, soda pop	Nonalcoholic, flavored, carbonated or non-carbonated beverages usually commercially prepared and sold in bottles or cans
Fruit drinks, punches, or ades	Sweetened beverages of diluted fruit juice
Sports drinks	Beverages designed to help athletes rehydrate, as well as replenish electrolytes, sugar, and other nutrients
Tea and coffee drinks:	Teas and coffees to which caloric sweeteners have been added
Energy drinks	Most energy drinks are carbonated drinks that contain large amounts of caffeine, sugar and other ingredients, such as vitamins, amino acids, and herbal stimulants
Sweetened milks or milk alternatives	Beverages prepared by blending sweetened powder or syrup and milk; the body's response to added sugar in milk may differ from that of other SSBs because of the presence of protein and other nutrients, adding sugar to milk substantially increases the calories per serving.

Several mechanisms have been advanced to explain how sugar directly and independently affects chronic disease risks. Bremer et al. (2011) and Nagai et al. (2009) postulated that, in the fed state, liver fructose increases lipogenesis, and reduces fatty acid oxidation, forming excessive liver fat and inflammation; this in turn inactivates the insulin signaling pathway, leading to hepatic insulin resistance. Sugary foods have been related to the development of insulin resistance in animal models. It has been proposed that reactive oxygen species, produced by Maillard reaction damages pancreatic beta cells, which ultimately results in insulin resistance, insulin secretion and overt diabetes (Teff et al., 2009; Santos et al., 2009; Hummasti and Hotamisligil, 2010).

Van Rompay et al. (2015) investigated characteristics associated with consumption of SSBs in a multi-ethnic sample of children/adolescents, and measured cross-sectional and longitudinal associations between SSB intake and plasma HDL cholesterol and triglycerides (TGs) over 12 months. Greater SSB consumption at baseline, and increased SSB intake during the study showed associations with blood lipids. Briefly, the investigators reported that intake of SSBs was positively associated with higher triglyceride (TG) concentrations among children and adolescents, and an inverse longitudinal association between SSB intake changes and HDL cholesterol changes, with decreased SSB intake associated with a greater increase in HDL cholesterol during the study.

Global Sugar Reduction Efforts

Sugar intake can be reduced by limiting the consumption SSBs and ASBs, which contain high amounts of sugars and by substituting fresh fruit and raw vegetables as snacks instead of sugary snacks. The WHO (2015) has strongly recommended that adults and children reduce the intake of free sugars to less than 10% of total energy intake.

Table 17. Nourishing Framework (WCRFI, 2015)

POLICY AREA	EVIDENCE FOR POLICY AREA	EXAMPLES OF POTENTIAL POLICY ACTIONS	
N	Nutrition label standards and regulations on the use of claims and implied claims on foods	The evidence suggests people who want to eat well use nutrient lists to choose healthier options. Interpretative labels help them when they find the labels hard to understand. Nutrition labels also create incentives for food manufacturers to reformulate their products, so helping populations more broadly by increasing the availability of foods of higher nutritional value. Clear standards are also needed on the use of nutrient and health claims. Evidence shows these claims alter the perception people have of these products – making it essential that they do not mislead.	e.g., Nutrient lists on food packages; clearly visible 'interpretive' and calorie labels; menu, shelf labels; rules on nutrient & health claims
O	Offer healthy foods and set standards in public institutions and other specific settings	We know from the evidence that making fruits and vegetables available in schools increases consumption. There is also evidence that food standards to restrict availability have the effect of reducing consumption of the restricted foods. For these actions to be effective for all children, they need to be sustained over time and accompanied by complementary behavior change communication techniques, such as "modeling," school gardens, and communication to all stakeholders involved in the provision and consumption of school food. Worksites and healthcare also present strong potential for improved eating among adults.	e.g., Fruit and vegetable programs; standards in education, work, health facilities; award schemes; choice architecture
U	Use economic tools to address food affordability and purchase incentives	Empirical estimates show that food prices influence, to a varying degree, how much food people buy. Targeted subsidies have been shown to help overcome affordability barriers to healthy foods for people on low incomes. Incentives, like financial rewards or price discounts, have also been shown to encourage people to switch to healthier options.	e.g., Targeted subsidies; price promotions at point of sale; unit pricing; health-related food taxes

POLICY AREA	EVIDENCE FOR POLICY AREA	EXAMPLES OF POTENTIAL POLICY ACTIONS	
		Emerging evidence from implemented taxes, as well as modelling studies, indicate the potential for effectiveness to reduce consumption. Given food choices are influenced by a whole host of factors, especially in modern, complex food markets, taxes must be designed very carefully to maximise effectiveness.	
R	Restrict food advertising and other forms of commercial promotion	There is clear evidence that the advertisements children see influence their food preferences and habits. There is also a lot of evidence that children and adolescents around the world are exposed to a whole host of other promotional techniques, whether it be on a billboard or through a phone or computer. Emerging evidence shows that restrictions work to reduce children's exposure of children to marketing, but this depends on the criteria used in the restrictions. Given the role played by parents and caregivers in what children eat, consideration is needed to how they are also influenced by promotional activities.	e.g., Restrict advertising to children that promotes unhealthy diets in all forms of media; sales promotions; packaging; sponsorship
I	Improve nutritional quality of the whole food supply	We are all influenced by the food that is available and affordable when we grow up, and the habits of the people around us. That's why people in different countries and communities consume differently. We know that when the food supply changes, so does what people eat. This is why we need to improve the quality of the food supply. Evidence from salt reduction indicates that people's tastes can change.	e.g., Reformulation to reduce salt and fats; elimination of trans fats; reduce energy density of processed foods; portion size limits
S	Set incentives and rules to create a healthy retail and food service environment	The neighborhood food environment – the retailers and other outlets where we buy our food – are the means through which people access the food supply. There is clear evidence that this environment influences the decisions we make about what we eat.	e.g., Incentives for shops to locate in underserved areas; planning restrictions on food outlets; in-store promotions

Table 17. (Continued)

POLICY AREA	EVIDENCE FOR POLICY AREA	EXAMPLES OF POTENTIAL POLICY ACTIONS	
H	Harness the food supply chain and actions across sectors to ensure coherence with health	Policies within this category aim to harness the whole food system, and the sectors which influence it, to ensure coherence with healthy eating. This is because the food system, and the policies that affect it, influence our food environment. What our food industry produces is in part a response to incentives in the supply chain. Sectors outside of health influence our ability to take policy action. Likewise, if governments implement policies contained in NOURISHING, they have repercussions upstream for the actors and activities in food systems. This wider relationship to the food supply chain presents an opportunity to support all the policies in NOURISHING with actions in the food supply chain.	e.g., Supply-chain incentives for production; public procurement through 'short' chains; health-in-all policies; governance structures for multi-sectorial engagement
I	Inform people about food and nutrition through public awareness	Awareness is one precursor to eating well. The evidence suggests that public campaigns can boost awareness. To influence consumption, they need to be sustained and use multiple channels.	e.g., Education about food-based dietary guidelines, mass media, social marketing; community and public information campaigns
N	Nutrition advice and counseling in health care settings	People with elevated risk factors for cancer and other non-communicable diseases – such as heavy bodyweight, high cholesterol or glucose intolerance –can benefit from advice provided by their health care provider. Such advice can also be given to people at low risk for prevention into the future. There is potentially a wide range of mechanisms for integrating nutrition advice into primary care, including counseling, self-help materials and computer-tailored messages. Randomized controlled trials suggest they can be effective if carefully designed and well-targeted. The most positive outcomes appear to be for people already at risk.	e.g., Nutrition advice for at-risk individuals; telephone advice and support; clinical guidelines for health professionals on effective interventions for nutrition

POLICY AREA	EVIDENCE FOR POLICY AREA	EXAMPLES OF POTENTIAL POLICY ACTIONS	
G	Give nutrition education and skills	The reason for nutrition education is to improve knowledge and the ability to put that knowledge into practice. Studies have demonstrated that nutrition knowledge and healthy dietary behavior are positively correlated. Higher levels of general education have been found to increase the ability of individuals to obtain and understand the health-related information needed to develop health-promoting behaviors. The evidence shows that interventions to provide education can be effective, but this depends on the pre-existing attitude, knowledge and habit strength of the targeted group. Education should thus be accompanied by changes in the food environments to effect longer-lasting change.	e.g., Nutrition, cooking/food production skills on education curricula; workplace health schemes; health literacy programs

This global network aims to monitor, benchmark and support actions to create healthy food environments, including through actions governing labeling, provision of foods in specific settings, prices, advertising and promotion, composition across the food supply, retail provision, and trade between countries. It has also developed a Government Healthy Food Environment Policy Index (Food-EPI) to assess the extent of government policy implementation against international best practice (WCRFI, 2015).

The American Heart Association has recommended a daily upper limit of 150 calories or nine teaspoons of sugar and 100 calories or six teaspoons of free sugar for men and women, respectively. The International Diabetes Federation (IDF) has proposed a framework for action on sugar with 12 measures to reduce sugar consumption (IDF, 2015).

The Centers for Disease Control (CDC), U.S. has recommended seven broad strategies for reducing SSB consumption (CDC, 2010). Levying a tax on SSBs has successfully reduced intake in other areas. For example, in 2014, Mexico added a 10% tax to drinks containing added sugar, which resulted in a 6% decline in purchases. A greater reduction of 9% was seen in low-income communities, where the risk of diabetes is higher. Similarly, consumption declined in France (3.1%), Hungary (6%) and Finland (3.1%) after taxes were introduced. More recently, Ford et al. (2015) examined the relation between beverage taxes and food and beverage purchases among U.S. households with a child 2–5 y of age and concluded that a tax on beverages high in sugar and/or fat may be associated with favorable changes in beverage purchases among US households with a preschool child. The researchers reported that price increases of 10, 15, and 20% on SSBs were related to fewer purchases of juice drinks. The WCRFI (2015) has developed a policy to assist governments in reducing the amount of sugar being consumed at a population level (Table 17). The policy can be used to help reduce sugar intake by influencing the availability, affordability, acceptability and awareness of sugar content in products.

Examples of Efforts to Reduce Population Sugar Consumption in Some Countries

1. U.S. - Healthy Beverage Executive Order (HBEO) (EO, 2011; Cradock et al., 2015)

Availability

To Eliminate the Sale of SSBs on City Property

The Healthy Beverage Executive Order (HBEO) was established by former Boston, Massachusetts, U.S. mayor Thomas M. Menino in 2011. The HBEO directed city departments to eliminate the sale of SSBs on city property and to adhere to the City of Boston's HBEO standards in vending machines and city-managed food or beverage services programs. The HBEO standards outlined the requirements for beverages that could be sold (EO, 2011). Calorically sweetened beverages, including some energy drinks, sports drinks, sweetened tea, and coffee drinks, were allowed if they contained ≤ 1 gram sugar/fluid ounce. These standards also addressed portion size for certain categories of beverages (e.g., milk, milk substitutes) and product mix (i.e., diet or other non-calorically sweetened beverages must make up no ≥ one-third of total offerings). Implementation consisted of "traffic-light signage" and educational materials at point of purchase.

The healthy beverage toolkit contained information about beverage standards and resources for implementing the HBEO requirements in Boston city agencies and other worksite settings in Boston. It also included point-of-decision consumer educational materials that used a traffic-light system to identify categories of beverages as shown in Table 18. City agencies were also provided with brochures, posters, and other promotional and education materials, which utilized the traffic-light identifiers (Boston Public Health Commission, 2011). Other opportunities included free workshops focused on the implementation of nutrition policy change, including such topics as working with contractors and vendors, technical assistance on legal issues, procurement policies, and special dietary needs Cradock et al. (2015) evaluated the impact of the HBEO on changes in beverage availability from March to September 2011 through March to November, 2013. They revealed that average beverage sugar grams and calories at access points decreased (sugar, −13.1 g; calories, −48.6 kcal; $p < .001$) following the implementation of the HBEO. The average proportion of high-sugar ("red") beverages available per access point declined (−27.8%, $p < .001$). City agencies were significantly more likely to sell only low-sugar beverages after the HBEO was implemented (OR = 4.88; 95% CI, 1.49–16.0).

Table 18. Boston Public Health Commission's point-of-purchase traffic-light classification system for beverages (Boston Public Health Commission, 2011; Cradock et al., 2015)

Beverage Color Classification	Criteria	Examples
Red: drink rarely, if at all	Over 12 g sugar per 12 oz.	• Regular soda • Energy drinks (regular) • Sports drinks (regular) • Pre-sweetened coffee and tea drinks • Juice drinks with added sugar • Whole or 2% milk
Yellow: drink occasionally	6 g to 12 g of sugar per 12 oz. or contains artificial sweeteners	• Diet soda • Diet iced tea • 100% fruit juice (in small portions) • Low-calorie sports drinks • Sweetened soymilk (in small portions) • Flavored 1% milk (in small portions) • Other low-sugar drinks • Energy drinks (artificially sweetened and/or containing ≤1 g sugar/oz) • Sports drinks (artificially sweetened and/or containing ≤1 g sugar/oz)
Green: drink plenty	0 to 5g of sugar per 12oz.	• Water • Seltzer water • 1% or skim milk (in small portions) • Unsweetened soymilk (in small portions)

Impact

The researchers concluded that community-wide access to healthier beverage alternatives can be promoted by policies such as the HBEO. Cradock and colleagues (2015) indicated that two years after the HBEO was issued, healthier beverage options were more accessible to city residents and employees in vending machines and in cafeterias and cafés on city properties. Also, city agencies were more likely to offer only healthier beverages for sale with no increase in beverage prices.

2. U.S. - The Zuni High School Diabetes Prevention Program (Ritenbaugh et al. 2003; CDC, 2013)

Availability

To Decrease SSB Consumption in Zuni High School

The Zuni High School Diabetes Prevention Program was a multicomponent intervention conducted among American Indian high school students in the U.S. Health education was provided to decrease SSB consumption and to increase knowledge of diabetes risk factors. The intervention was combined with environmental change to increase access to potable drinking water and physical activity. Evaluation was done at baseline, 1.5, and 3 years.

Impact

The findings demonstrated that by the third year, the 400 students of Zuni High School consumed almost no sugared soft drinks at school, a decrease from 800 12-ounce cans/week/400 students (24 ounces/week/student). Soft drinks had been replaced by 150 gallons of water weekly from the water coolers (24 ounces/week/student) and 260 12-ounce cans of diet soda (7.8 ounces/week/student).

3. Australia: Queensland's "Smart Choices, the Healthy Food and Drink Supply Strategy (WCRFI, 2015)

Availability

Reducing the Availability of Sugary Products in Schools

Smart Choices, the Healthy Food and Drink Supply Strategy for Queensland Schools is all about offering healthy food and drink choices to students in Queensland schools. Its implementation is mandatory in state schools and strongly encouraged in non-state schools. Foods and drinks have been classified into three categories according to their nutritional value: green, amber and red (Table 19).

Impact

The Smart Choices, the Healthy Food and Drink Supply Strategy for Queensland Schools - launched in 2005 and became mandatory in all state schools in 2007. It was implemented in almost all tuckshops/canteens (96-99%). Tuckshops/canteens (97%) reported all red foods have been removed, while 91% reported increased availability of green foods. The strategy effectively reduced the availability of unhealthy foods on school premises, especially SSBs (WCRFI, 2015).

Table 19. Under Smart Choices, foods and drinks have been classified into three categories according to their nutritional value: Green, Amber and Red

GREEN 'Have plenty' Encourage and promote these smart choices	AMBER 'Select carefully' Do not let these foods and drinks dominate the choices and avoid large serving sizes	RED 'Occasionally' Not to be supplied on more than two occasions per term
GREEN foods and drinks are typically fresh or minimally processed. These foods and drinks are:: • excellent sources of important nutrients • low in saturated fat and/or added sugar and/or added salt • less likely to result in excess energy intake and reduce the risk of weight gain GREEN foods and drinks should be promoted to students as the best available choice and should dominate the daily canteen menu	AMBER foods and drinks have had some sugar, salt or fat added during processing. These foods and drinks: • have some nutritional value • have moderate amounts of saturated fat and/or added sugar and/or added salt • can contribute to excess energy intake and weight gain AMBER foods and drinks should not dominate the menu at the expense of healthier GREEN choices. If selecting AMBER foods and drinks, consider offering them only on certain days of the week and use small serving sizes.	RED foods and drinks are highly processed and have added sugar, salt or fat. These foods and drinks: • lack nutritional value • are high in saturated fat and/or added sugar and/ or added salt • can contribute to excess energy intake and weight gain RED foods and drinks should not be supplied by the school on more than two occasions per term. Refer to the 'Occasional' RED food and drink criteria tables to determine if a food or drink fits into the RED category

Available at: http://education.qld.gov.au

4. Netherlands - Healthy Logo: Netherlands 'Choices' Logo (WCRFI, 2015)

Reducing the Availability of Sugar in the Food Supply: Product Reformulation

On the basis of criteria that define maximum levels of nutrients as added sugar, salt and fat products are entitled to carry the Choices logo on the front of the package (FoP). The green stamp with healthy choice represents the healthy choice within a category of basic products. These basic products – including bread, milk, fruit and vegetables – are essential to a healthy diet. The blue stamp with conscious choice helps to select healthier options within non-basic product categories, including soups, sauces and snacks. These logos emphasize the positive nutritional aspects to consumers as no products are presented in a negative frame.

Impact

Most products carrying the logo have been reformulated to meet the logo's criteria, including soups, sandwiches and processed meat. Saturated fat, added sugars and calories have been significantly reduced in dairy products to meet the logo criteria and added sugar has been reduced in sauces. New products specifically formulated to meet the criteria were developed following the launch of the logo – typically, snacks; processed fruits and vegetables; fruit juices and drinks; and soups.

5. France - The French Soda Tax (Berardi et al., 2012)

Affordability

Reducing Affordability of Sugary Drinks

The tax, comprising approximately of 11 euro cents (US$0.12) for a 1.5 L soda, came into effect 2012. It is a mandatory excise tax to be paid to the government by the producers or sellers, which will be passed on to the consumer by price increase of the product.

Impact

The tax significantly increased the price of taxable beverages (e.g., soda, fruit drinks and flavored waters). Six months after implementation, the tax was shifted 100% to soda prices, but only 60 and 85% to fruit drinks and flavored water, respectively.

Other National Examples

In Ecuador, a regulation of the Ministry of Public Health requires packaged foods to carry a "traffic light" label in which the levels of fats, sugar, and salt are indicated by red (high), orange (medium), or green (low). This was implemented in 2014 (IFPRI, 2015). In Costa Rica, Executive Decree No. 36910-MEP-S permits schools to sell only food and drink that meet specific nutritional criteria. This was implemented in 2012 according to IFPRI, 2015. In 2008, the Iranian Ministries of Education and Health developed the Guidelines for Healthy Diet and School Buffets. In 2013 the nutrition part of the guidelines was updated. The guidelines list foods based on their sugar, salt, fat, and additive content (IFPRI, 2015).

Fats, Cholesterol and Chronic Disease

Fats are a family of compounds comprised mainly of carbon and hydrogen with a small amount of oxygen. The major fat in food is triglyceride, a molecule of glycerol with three fatty acids attached (Figure 24). Fats are insoluble in water and fatty acids come in a variety of sizes. However, all fat in foods contain a mixture of different fatty acids. Fatty acids also carry different number of hydrogen atoms per carbon atom (Figure 24).

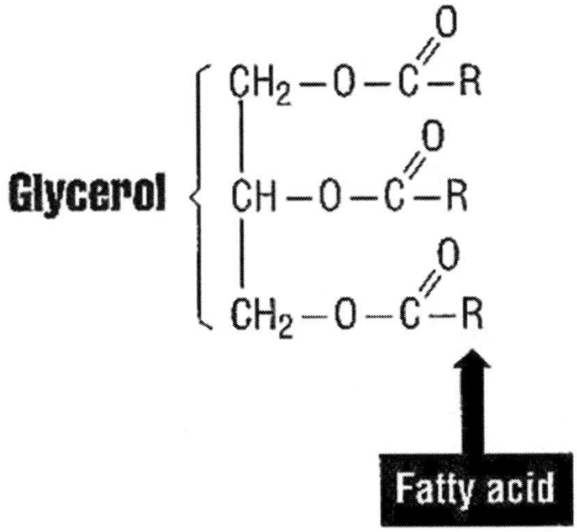

Figure 24. A triglyceride. The "R" represents fatty acids chemically bound to the glycerol (Woteki and Thomas (1992).

Figure 25a shows a saturated fatty acid, which has the maximum number of hydrogen atoms (two) attached to every carbon atom, except for those on each end. In other words, the molecule is "saturated" with hydrogen atoms. Fats high in saturated fatty acids are usually solid at room and refrigeration temperatures. Inspecting Figure 25b, there are two hydrogen atoms missing in the middle of the molecule, one from each of two adjoining carbon atoms (an unsaturation). Such fats are called monounsaturated fatty acids (MUFAs). Figure 25c and d are missing more hydrogen atoms, from adjacent pairs of carbon atom (polyunsaturation). Fatty acids with more than one unsaturation are called polyunsaturated fatty acids (PUFAs). Fats with a large percentage of MUFAs and PUFAs are typically liquids. It is worth noting that PUFAs are further classified by where the unsaturations occur in the fatty acid molecule. For example, Eicosapentaenoic acid (EPA) (Figure 26) is one of the main omega-3 fatty acids in fish oil. This means that the first unsaturation occurs at the third carbon atom from the omega end of the fatty acid (the end with three hydrogen atoms). It can be seen then why linoleic and linolenic acids are called omega-6 and omega-3 fatty acids, respectively (Figure 25c and d).

Cholesterol is found in animal source foods (egg yolk, liver, meat, some types of shellfish, and whole milk dairy products). The structure of cholesterol is shown in Figure 27. Cholesterol is endogenous in the body as an important component of several tissues, especially the brain and nervous system (Woteki and Thomas, 1992). The functions of cholesterol include the production of bile acids, various hormones, and vitamin D.

Cholesterol moves through the blood in clusters of molecules made of fat and protein called lipoproteins. Most of the cholesterol in the body is carried by three types of lipoproteins: high-density lipoprotein (HDL), low-density lipoprotein (LDL), and very-low-density lipoprotein (VLDL). Cholesterol found in HDL is called HDL-cholesterol, and cholesterol found in LDL is called LDL-cholesterol (Woteki and Thomas, 1992). The sum of HDL-, LDL-, and VLDL-cholesterol in the blood stream is usually referred to as the total serum cholesterol.

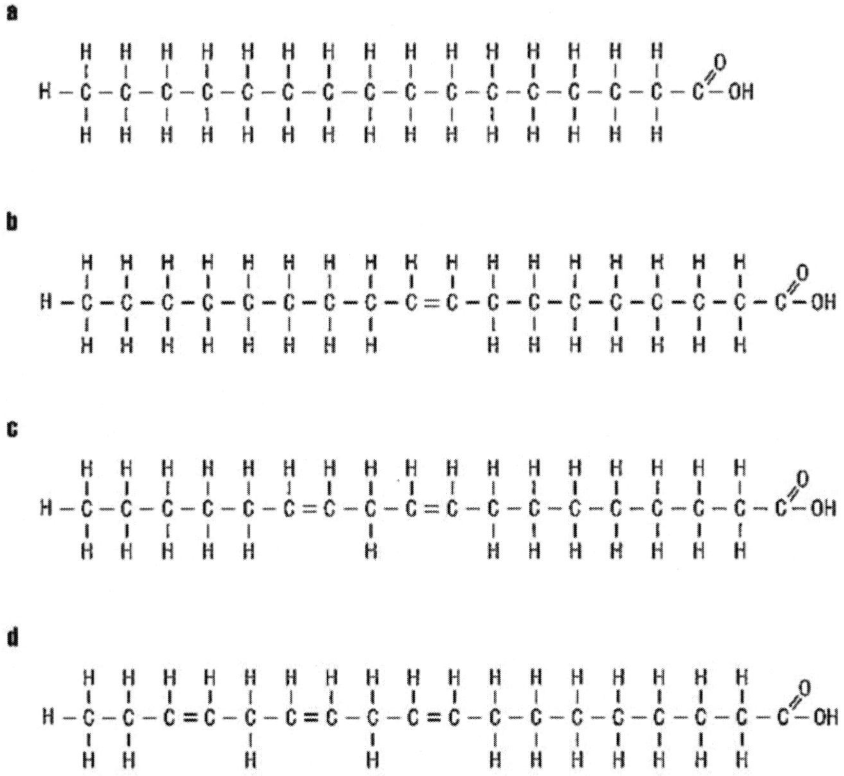

Figure 25. Comparison of the structure of four fatty acids: (a) palmitic, (b) oleic, (c) linoleic, and (d) linolenic acids (Woteki and Thomas (1992).

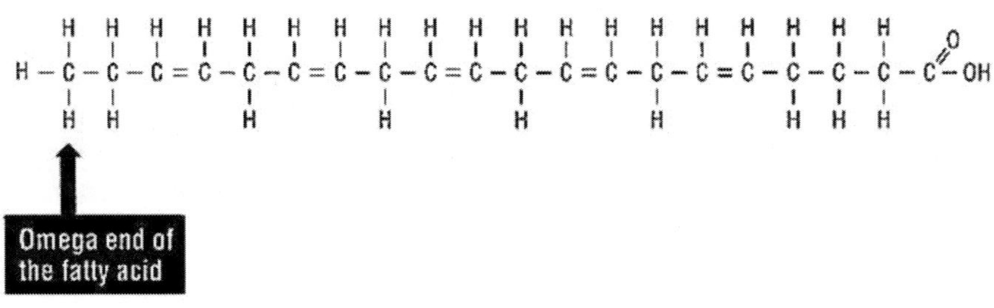

Figure 26. Eicosapentaenoic acid, an omega-3 fatty acid (Woteki and Thomas (1992).

Elevated serum cholesterol is a major cause of disease burden in both the developed and developing world, which increases the risks of heart diseases and stroke. However, elevated serum cholesterol is a modifiable risk factor. Globally, 33% of ischemic heart disease is attributable to elevated serum cholesterol (WHO, 2010). Overall, raised cholesterol is estimated to cause 2.6 million deaths (4.5% of total) and 29.7 million disability adjusted life years (DALYS) (WHO, 2010). Cholesterol-lowering initiatives include reduced dietary intake of saturated fats and cholesterol, weight control, and increased physical activity.

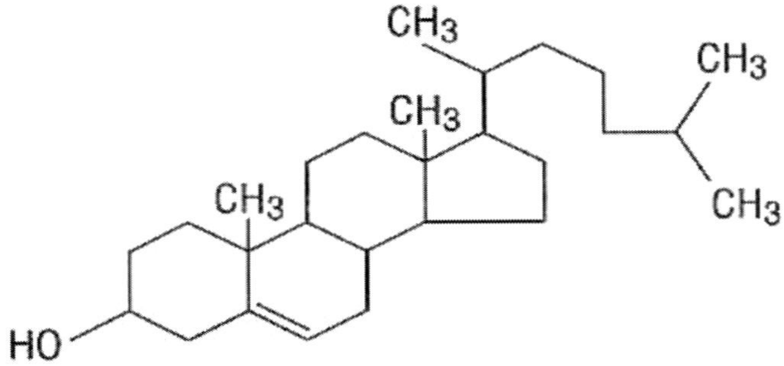

Figure 27. Cholesterol (Woteki and Thomas (1992).

According to the World Health Organization (2010), a 10% reduction in serum cholesterol in males aged 40 has been reported to result in a 50% reduction in heart disease within 5 years. Similarly, a 10% reduction in serum cholesterol reduction for men aged 70 years can result in an average 20% reduction in heart disease occurrence in the next 5 years (WHO, 2010). In Ireland, a 30% reduction in the heart disease death rate has been attributed to 4.6% reduction of the mean total cholesterol for the population. In Finland, 50% of the decline in ischemic heart disease mortality has been explained by the reduction of population blood cholesterol level.

Venkitachalam et al. (2012) concluded from a global study of outpatients at high risk of atherothrombosis that persistent elevated total cholesterol was more likely among people living in countries with lower GNI, higher out-of-pocket healthcare costs, and less efficient healthcare systems. The global prevalence of elevated total serum cholesterol (≥ 5.0 mmol/L) among adults was 39% in 2008. WHO African and South East Asian Regions showed the lowest percentages of elevated cholesterol, 22.6 and 29.0%, respectively (WHO, 2012).

Preventive Care

It has been established that serum cholesterol levels can be lowered by consumption of a balanced diet, regular physical activity and maintenance of optimal weight. Several strategies have been suggested to limit cholesterol consumption.

1. Dietary guidelines to lower cholesterol

- Limit the intake of saturated and trans fats, consuming no more than 10% of daily calories from saturated fat, and the avoidance of trans fats. It is estimated that a 2% increase in energy intake from trans fats increases the incidence of heart disease by 23%.
- Consume more whole grains, whole wheat bread and pasta, oatmeal, oat bran, and brown rice.
- Increase intake of fruits and vegetables, which are high in fiber and can help lower cholesterol levels. Studies have shown that plant-based diets are associated with up to 15% decreases in total cholesterol and LDL cholesterol. The Stepwise approach to surveillance (STEPS) survey is a standardized WHO chronic disease risk factor instrument. Over the past 10 years, STEPS was utilized in 30 sub-Saharan African countries (SSA). The findings indicated that 89% of those surveyed did not consume

the recommended five daily servings of fruits and vegetables (The Economist Intelligence Unit, 2014).
- Limit cholesterol in your diet. The highest amounts are found in egg yolks, whole milk products, and organ meats.
- Consume fatty fish, at least two servings per week.
- Eat phytosterols and stanols found in nuts, seeds, vegetable oils, and fortified food products, such as orange juice, yogurt, and salad dressing. Studies show that eating 2 to 3 grams of phytosterols daily reduces total cholesterol by up to 11% and LDL cholesterol by up to 15%.
- Increase intake of high fiber foods

2. The recommendation

- Grains: 6 to 8 servings per day (50% should be whole grains)
- Vegetables: 3 to 5 servings per day
- Fruits: 4 to 5 servings per day
- Fat-free or low-fat dairy: 2 to 3 servings per day
- Lean meat, poultry, seafood: 3 to 6 oz. per day (about the size of a deck of cards)
- Fats and oils: 2 to 3 tbsp. per day (use unsaturated fats)
- Nuts, seeds, legumes: 3 to 5 servings per week
- Sweets, sugars: 5 or fewer servings per week (the fewer, the better)
- Restrict sodium (salt, including salt already added to food) to less than 2,400 mg per day)
- Limit alcohol intake to one and drinks per day for women and men, respectively
- The therapeutic lifestyle changes diet is recommended for people who have high cholesterol. With the TLC diet, less than 7% of your daily total calories should come from saturated fat, and only 25% to 35% of your daily calories should come from fat, overall. Sodium should be limited to 2,400 mg per day
- The Mediterranean style diet concentrates on whole grains, fresh fruits and vegetables, fish, olive oil, and moderate, daily wine consumption. This diet is low in saturated fat, but high in monounsaturated fat. It is naturally rich in fiber, antioxidants, and omega-3 fatty acids and appears to be heart healthy: In a long-term study of 423 people who had a heart attack, those who followed a Mediterranean style diet had a 50 to 70% lower risk of recurrent heart disease compared with people who received no special dietary counseling.

3. Maintaining healthy weight

- Being overweight increases the risk of high cholesterol and heart disease. Even a 5 to 10 pound weight loss can lower LDL twice as much as diet alone. Weight loss often results in lower triglyceride levels and increased HDL, too.

4. Physical activity

- Regular physical activity reduces the risk of death from heart disease and helps lower LDL cholesterol levels, especially when combined with a healthy diet. Thirty minutes of moderate exercise five times per week can help with weight loss or maintenance, reduce LDL and triglyceride levels, and increase levels of HDL. It has been shown that every 10 minutes of added physical activity per session is associated with a 1.4 mg/dL increase in HDL cholesterol. Physical activity may also lower blood pressure.

High blood cholesterol includes hyperlipidaemia, which refers to a high concentration of all the different blood fats (also called lipids) in the blood. The consumption of large quantities of food with high levels of saturated and trans fatty acids and foods high in cholesterol, results in high blood cholesterol levels, which increases the risk of a heart attack (Steyn, 2006). Too little fiber in the diet also contributes to high blood cholesterol.

Lowering cholesterol level reduces your risk of heart disease and stroke. It has been shown that for every 1% reduction in cholesterol levels there is a 2% reduction in the rate of heart disease. Individuals with heart disease or are at higher risk benefit most from lowering their cholesterol. Changes in lifestyle, improved diet and more physical activity, are the most effective means of both preventing and, in less severe cases, treating high LDL cholesterol levels. Table 20 shows the recommended targets for cholesterol levels. A summary of life's simple seven goals from the AHA is shown in Table 21. Shown below is an example of Argentina, which has implemented a policy to improve the nutritional quality of foods produced by food processors. It is a nationwide policy to reduce fat and cholesterol in foods.

Table 20. European and American recommended targets for cholesterol levels

	Europe (mmol/L and mg/dL)	United States
Optimal Total Cholesterol	≤5.0 mmol/L or less	5.1 mmol/L
LDL Cholesterol	3.0 mmol/L or less	2.6 mmol/L or less
HDL Cholesterol	1.2 mmol/L or more in women 1.0 mmol/L in men	≥ 2.6 mmol/L
Triglycerides	1.7 mmol/L or less	1.7 mmol/L or less

Table 21. Summary of life's simple seven goals from the AHA (American Heart Association)

Lifestyle Behavior/Risk Factor	American Heart Association (AHA) Goal
Nonsmoking	Smoking abstinence, smoking cessation
Regular physical activity	At least 150 minutes of moderate intensity or 75 minutes of vigorous intensity each week
Healthy diet*	4.5 or more cups of fruit/vegetables daily; 2 or more 3.5-oz servings of fish/wk; ≤450 kcal of sugar-sweetened beverages/week; 3 or more 1-oz servings of fiber-rich whole grains/day; <1500 g sodium/day
Healthy body weight	Body mass index (BMI) <25 kg/m^2
Non-drug treated total cholesterol level	<200 mg/dL
Non-drug treated blood pressure Non-drug treated fasting glucose level	<120/80 mm Hg <100 mg/dL

* In the context of a diet that is appropriate in energy balance, pursuing an overall dietary pattern that is consistent with a DASH (dietary approaches to stop hypertension) - type eating plan, including but not limited to these 5 dietary goals.

Argentina's Strategy to Reduce Fat and Cholesterol Intake

Mandatory Removal of Trans Fat in Foods

In 2010, the Argentine Food Code was amended to limit trans fat content to <2% of total vegetable fats in oils and margarines and 5% of total fat in all other foods (implemented in 2014) (IFPRI, 2015)

Physical Activity

Physical activity (PA) and exercise are now considered principal interventions for use in primary and secondary prevention of chronic diseases (Durstine et al., 2013). Physical inactivity has been linked to increased levels of obesity, some types of cancer and other types of chronic diseases (Kreuger et al., 2002; 23 Hardman, 2001). These conditions are drastically improved or prevented when PA and exercise are part of a preventive and management plan (Durstine et al., 2013). PA has been recognized as one lifestyle shift, which is partly responsible for the earlier onset of chronic disease (Blair and Brodney, 1999). Lee et al. (2012) have estimated that in 2008, physical inactivity was responsible for 6, 7, 10 and 10% of CHD, T2D, breast and colon cancers, respectively. The researchers concluded that if inactivity was decreased instead by 10 or 25%, more than 533,000 and more than 1·3 million deaths, respectively, could be averted every year (Lee et al., 2012). It has been demonstrated that moderate amounts of physical activity can help to reduce various chronic diseases related to lifestyle (Kolbe-Alexander, 2006). Data from a comparative study of 51 countries showed that 47.6 and 44.7% of women and men, respectively, were physically inactive (Guthold et al., 2008). An older 2002 South African Youth Risk Behaviour Survey revealed a similar pattern among young people. It revealed that 43 and 30.5% of females and males, respectively, participated in insufficient or no physical activity (Reddy et al., 2002). The STEPS data show that only a minority of Africans engage in vigorous physical activity. An older study conducted in the urban and rural settings of Cameroon and Tanzania concluded that physical inactivity was associated with chronic diseases such as obesity, diabetes, and hypertension (Sobngwi et al., 2002). Levitt et al. (1999) reported an independent association between low levels of physical activity and type 2 diabetes in a poor, peri-urban community near Cape Town, South Africa. In a study conducted in Iran by Shokrvash et al. (2013) among adolescents, both female and male students did not meet the recommended physical activity times for adolescents (60 minutes of moderate/vigorous physical activity/day). The reprinted abstract shows the state of physical activity in selected African countries.

Physical Activity in 22 African Countries: Results from the World Health Organization Stepwise Approach to Chronic Disease Risk Factor Surveillance (Guthold et al., 2011)

Background

Baseline physical activity data are needed to effectively plan programs and policies to prevent non-communicable diseases, but for many African countries these data are lacking.

Purpose

The purpose was to describe and compare levels and patterns of physical activity among adults across 22 African countries.

Methods

Data from 57,038 individuals from 22 countries (11 national and 11 subnational samples) that participated in the STEPwise approach to chronic disease risk factor surveillance (2003–2009) were analyzed in 2010. The validated Global Physical Activity Questionnaire (GPAQ) was used to assess days and duration of physical activity at work, for transport, and during leisure time in a typical week.

Results

Overall, 83.8% of men and 75.7% of women met WHO physical activity recommendations (at least 150 minutes of moderate activity per week or equivalent). Country prevalence ranged from 46.8% (Mali) to 96.0% (Mozambique). Physical activity, both at work and for transport, including walking, had large contributions to overall physical activity, while physical activity during leisure time was rare in the analyzed countries.

Conclusion

Physical activity levels varied greatly across African countries and population subgroups. Leisure time activity was consistently low. These data will be useful to inform policymakers and to guide interventions to promote physical activity.

WHO's Global Recommendation On Physical Activity For Health

- Recommended levels of physical activity for health 5–17 years old:
    - Children and young people aged 5–17 years old should accumulate at least 60 minutes of moderate to vigorous-intensity physical activity daily.
    - Physical activity of amounts greater than 60 minutes daily will provide additional health benefits.
    - Most of daily physical activity should be aerobic. Vigorous-intensity activities should be incorporated, including those that strengthen muscle and bone, at least three times weekly.
- Recommended levels of physical activity for health for adults 18-64 years old
    - Adults aged 18–64 years should do at least 150 minutes of moderate-intensity aerobic physical activity throughout the week, or do at least 75 minutes of vigorous-intensity aerobic physical activity throughout the week, or an equivalent combination of moderate- and vigorous-intensity activity.
    - Aerobic activity should be performed in bouts of at least 10 minutes duration
    - For additional health benefits, adults should increase their moderate-intensity aerobic physical activity to 300 minutes per week, or engage in 150 minutes of vigorous-intensity aerobic physical activity per week, or an equivalent combination of moderate- and vigorous-intensity activity.

  - Muscle-strengthening activities should be done involving major muscle groups on two or more days per week.
- Recommended levels of physical activity for health for adults 65 years old and above:
  - Adults aged 65 years and above should do at least 150 minutes of moderate-intensity aerobic physical activity throughout the week, or do at least 75 minutes of vigorous-intensity aerobic physical activity throughout the week, or an equivalent combination of moderate- and vigorous-intensity activity.
  - Aerobic activity should be performed in bouts of at least 10 minutes duration.
  - For additional health benefits, adults aged 65 years and above should increase their moderate intensity aerobic physical activity to 300 minutes per week, or engage in 150 minutes of vigorous intensity aerobic physical activity per week, or an equivalent combination of moderate- and vigorous intensity activity.
  - Adults of this age group with poor mobility should perform physical activity to enhance balance and prevent falls on three or more days per week.
  - Muscle-strengthening activities should be done involving major muscle groups, on two or more days a week.
  - When adults of this age group cannot do the recommended amounts of physical activity due to health conditions, they should be as physically active as their abilities and conditions allow.

Examples of Efforts to Increase Physical Activity Levels (PAL)

1. New Zealand - The Green Prescription (GRx)

The initiative consists of two components: GRx (for adults) and the GRx Active Families program, which aims to increase physical activity for children, young people and their families. GRx and GRx Active Families were introduced in 1998 and 2004, respectively. It targets physically inactive people seeking primary health care. In 2013, the GRx budget was allocated additional funds for the next four years to increase adult referrals, especially for those with pre-diabetes or diabetes. A brief consultation with a primary care professional involves a discussion on the benefits of increased physical activity and joint agreement on goals (Figure 28). The agreed goal is then "prescribed" to the patient on green paper and faxed to the local sports foundation. Exercise specialists follow up with at least three telephone calls and the participant receives quarterly newsletters outlining opportunities for activity with the foundation.

Impact

An increase of 975 kcal/week in total energy expenditure among those in the intervention group was observed, and an increase in leisure energy expenditure of 247 kcal/week. Leisure time minutes of physical activity have also increased by 33.6 minutes per week, and those in the intervention group report an increased feelings of well-being. GRx has been shown to be effective in changing physical activity behavior and self-reported quality of life, and is cost-effective (MOH, 2015).

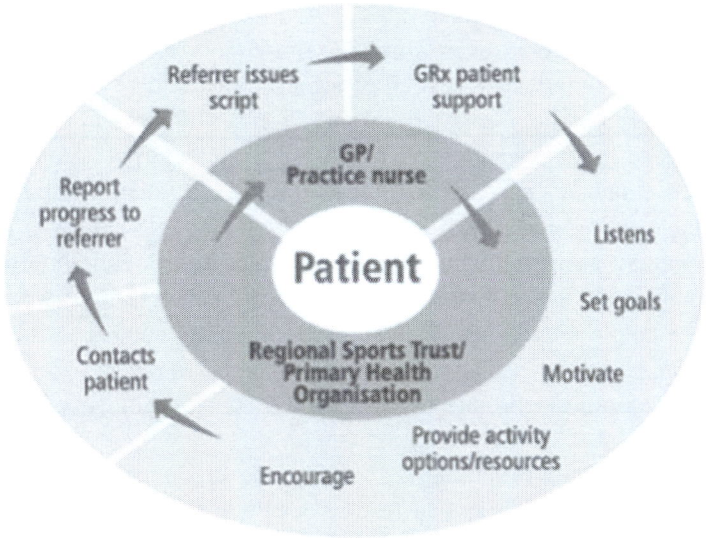

Figure 28. How the Green Prescription (GRx) process works for the health professional and patient.

2. South Africa - The Community Health Intervention Program (CHIPs) (Kolbe-Alexander et al., 2006).

The initiative for older adults was a twice per week, peer-led physical activity classes in disadvantaged communities in rural South Africa. The classes took place following existing meetings of community seniors over a 20- week period.

Impact

CHIPs has been classified as moderately effective. Significant improvements were seen in dynamic balance, lower body strength, and systolic blood pressure. This program has been running, using a community development model through peer-leadership, for over seven years.

3. U.S. - Active Choices and Active Living Every Day (Wilcox et al., 2006)

Wilcox et al. (2006) evaluated the effects of 2 evidence-based physical activity interventions on self-reported physical activity and related outcomes in midlife and older adults. Four community-based organizations implemented Active Choices, a 6-month, telephone-based program, and five implemented Active Living Every Day, a 20-week, group-based program. Both programs emphasized behavioral skills necessary to become more physically active. Participants completed pretest and posttest surveys.

Impact

Participants (n=838) were mostly women with an average of 68.4 ±9.4 years. Posttest surveys were returned by 72% of the participants. Statistically significant increases in moderate-to-vigorous physical activity and total physical activity, decreases in depressive symptoms and stress, increases in satisfaction with body appearance and function, and decreases in BMI were reported. The first year of Active for Life demonstrated that Active Choices and Active Living Every Day, 2 evidence-based physical activity programs, can be successfully translated into community settings with diverse populations. Additionally, the magnitudes of change in outcomes were similar to those reported in the efficacy trials.

National efforts are underway in several countries to manipulate two of the most common modifiable risk factors for the escalating chronic disease dilemma in the world (unhealthy diets and physical inactivity). Reducing salt intake has been identified as one of the most cost-effective measures countries can take to improve population health outcomes. Over time, some countries have successfully initiated salt reduction strategies to lower the incidence of CVD. Some strategies utilized include: consumer education, food industry partnerships, intervention in public settings, FoL, legislative strategies and food reformulation. Strategies reported have been both voluntary and mandatory. Developing countries still need to develop national salt reduction strategies. They should be guided by the WHO global action plan for the prevention and control of chronic diseases, which contains suggested policy options for salt reduction.

The literature abounds with strategies, policies and recommendations for reducing the intake of SSBs; especially as it is linked to diabetes. Several global sugar reduction efforts have been described in this chapter. The NOURISHING Framework (Table17) outlines the evidence for policy area and gives several examples of potential policy actions. The CDC has recommended seven broad categories for reducing SSB consumption. Levying a tax on SSBs, eliminating the sale of SSBs in schools, city/state/federal property, product formulation have proven to be very effective and low-cost strategies, which could be easily implemented in developing countries.

Elevated serum cholesterol is a major cause of disease burden, which increases the risk of HD and stroke. Cholesterol lowering initiatives include reduced intake of saturated fats, trans fat, cholesterol-rich foods, weight control, and increased physical activity. Several strategies, including intake of a balanced diet, regular physical activity and maintenance of healthy weight can lower cholesterol levels. Nationwide policy to reduce fat and cholesterol in foods has been initiated in Argentina, for example.

WHO has global recommendations on physical activity for health for member countries. Only a minority of Africans engage in vigorous physical activity. The same is true for Iran. Efforts are underway in some countries, such as New Zealand, South Africa and the U.S. to increase physical activity levels. A variety of cost-effective chronic disease interventions have been documented for all regions of the world, including sub-Saharan Africa. Each country, regardless of the level of its resources, has the potential to make significant improvements in chronic disease prevention and control, and to take steps towards achieving the global goal. Indeed, resources are necessary, but a large amount can be achieved for little cost, for example altering diets and increasing physical activity.

Chapter 7

Chronic Diseases and Climate Change

Connecting Chronic Diseases and Climate Change

The two most demanding modern global public health threats are climate change and chronic diseases (Briggs et al., 2013; Webb and Egger, 2013). Globally, climate change is a major threat to the health of populations in both rural and urban areas (WHO, 2009). Rising global temperatures are projected to alter disease patterns, increase food and water insecurity, and lead to extreme climatic events (Costello et al., 2009). At first glance, the connection between climate change and chronic diseases appears unrelated, except for their coexistence as major threats to global health and sustainability. However, growing evidence points to a linkage between chronic diseases and climate change. It is important to note that the impact of climate change on human health dealt with in this book is not all-encompassing. The intent is to raise awareness about climate change and its relationship to human health in general and chronic diseases in particular.

The effects of climate change on health are likely to be predominantly negative and impact most heavily on developing countries where the capacity to adapt is weakest. Simply put, climate change refers to the average increasing global temperature. The mean global temperature increase ranges from 1.8 to 4.0ºC, while the estimated average increase by 2100 is 30ºC (IPCC, 2007). Put another way, the term climate change describes long-term changes in the statistical distribution of weather patterns over specific time periods. The duration of the time period could range from decades to millions of years. The changes could occur in the average weather conditions or in the distribution of weather events. The International Energy Agency (iea) defines climate change as the change in climate (regional temperature, precipitation, extreme weather, etc.) caused by increase in the greenhouse effect (GHE). GHE is the process where greenhouse gases, such as water vapor, CO_2 and methane in the atmosphere, absorb and re-emit heat being released from the earth, while trapping warmth. Greenhouse gases absorb infrared radiation (heat) (http://www.iea.org).

The intergovernmental panel on climate change (IPCC) refers to climate change as an alteration in the state of the climate, which can be recognized (for example, using statistical tests) by variations in the mean and/or the inconsistency of its properties. Usually these changes, which are attributable to natural variability or a result of human activity, persist for an extended period such as decades or longer. On the other hand, the United Nations

Framework of Convention on Climate Change used the term to describe a change of climate attributable to human activity, which alters the composition of the global atmosphere, in addition to natural climate variability observed over comparable time periods. Figure 29 shows some of the complex ecological networks that can be disrupted by climate change and the human health implications of these disruptions. Figure 30 shows a simpler schematic of the three primary pathways by which climate change affects health.

Although climate change impacts the world, developing countries are expected to bear the brunt of the burden. Some of the effects of climate change include higher temperatures, rising sea levels, more droughts, strong storms and heat waves. Developing countries already account for more than 50% of total carbon emissions (Figure 31). For example, Brazil produces more CO_2 per head than Germany. The Economist cited a 2006 report, which calculated the cost of a 2°C rise in global temperature as equivalent to 1% of world GDP (The Economist, 2009). However, in its 2010 World Development Report, the World Bank revised these estimates to indicate that the cost to Africa and South Asia will be more like 4 to 5% (World Bank, 2010). It is predicted that developing countries would bear 80% of the climate change burden.

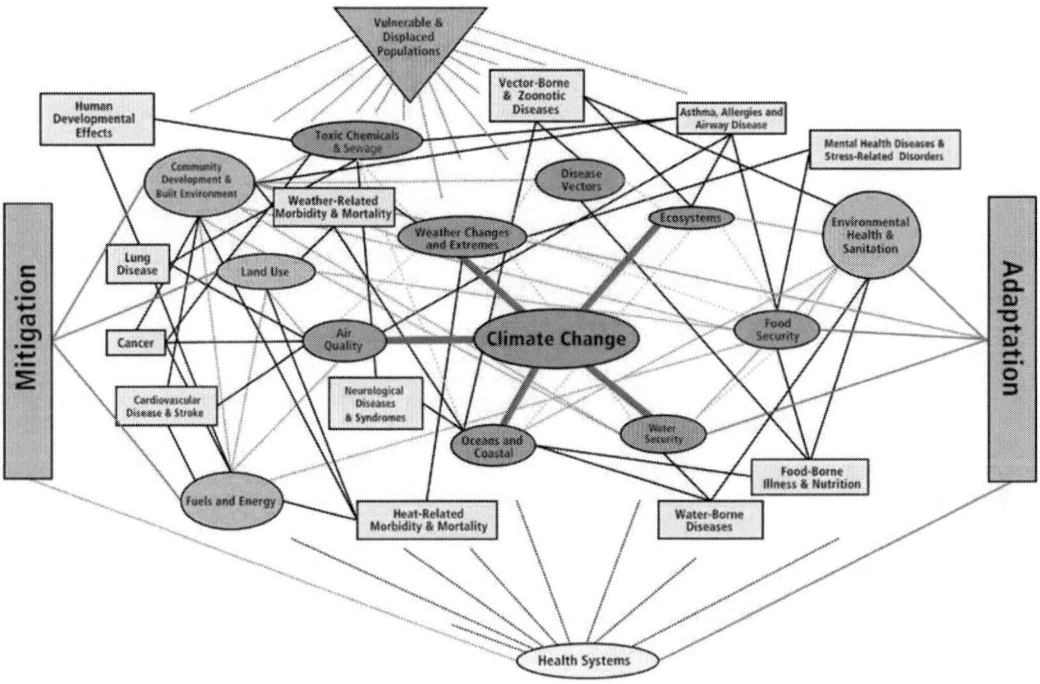

Figure 29. Climate change and human health - "Climate change has direct impacts on five aspects of the human environment (red lines, purple circles) that in turn impact additional environmental factors. These environmental changes then alter 12 separate aspects of human health (in boxes). Mitigation and adaptation alter the human environment in order to address climate change and, in this way, alter human health. Finally, susceptible populations exist for all climate-targeted health points, and the health systems play an integral role in addressing the health concerns driven by climate change" (Portier et al., 2010).

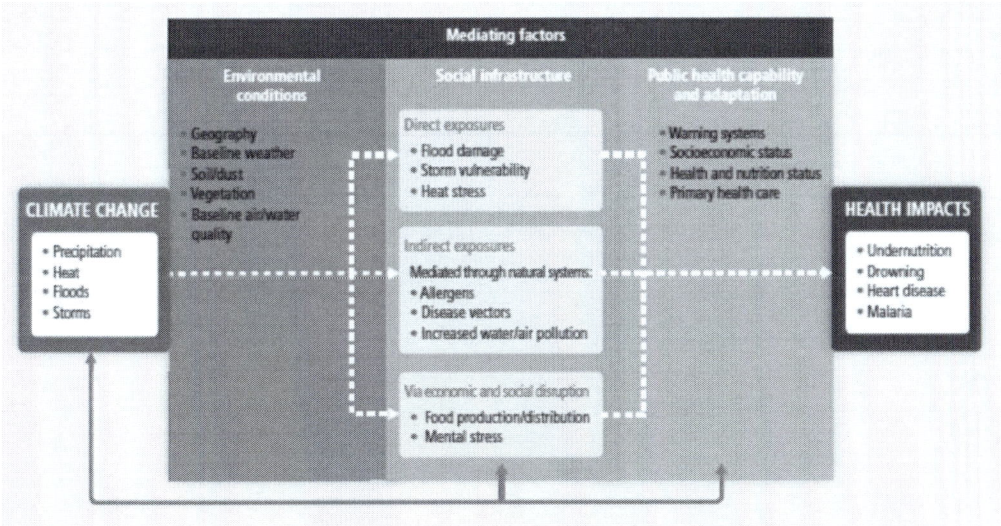

Figure 30. Conceptual diagram showing three primary pathways by which climate change affects health (Smith et al. 2014).

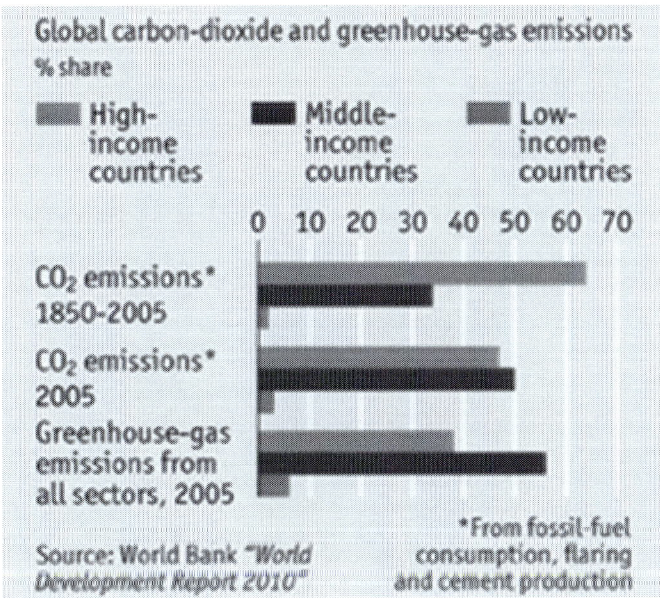

Figure 31. Global CO_2 and greenhouse-gas emissions (World Bank "World Development Report 2010").

Climate Change and Health in Context

Higher incidences of climate-related, chronic disease represent increasing challenges to vulnerable populations such as the poor and elderly (Balbus and Malina, 2009; Smith et al., 2014). Table 22 shows a three-way classification and causal pathway for categories of climate change risks to health taken from Butler and Harley (2010). The cost of global warming is also escalating. As shown in Figure 32, older data have indicated that in 1981-1985 and 2001-2005, less than 500 million and 1.5 billion people, respectively, required international disaster-assistance. In 2000, the World Health Organization reported that climate change caused a loss of 5.5 million disability-adjusted life years (DALYs) or healthy years of life lost; most of it in Africa and Asia. Between 2030 and 2050, the number of additional deaths attributable to climate change annually is expected to be 250,000; and the direct damage costs to health are estimated to be between US$2 to 4 bn. per year by 2030.

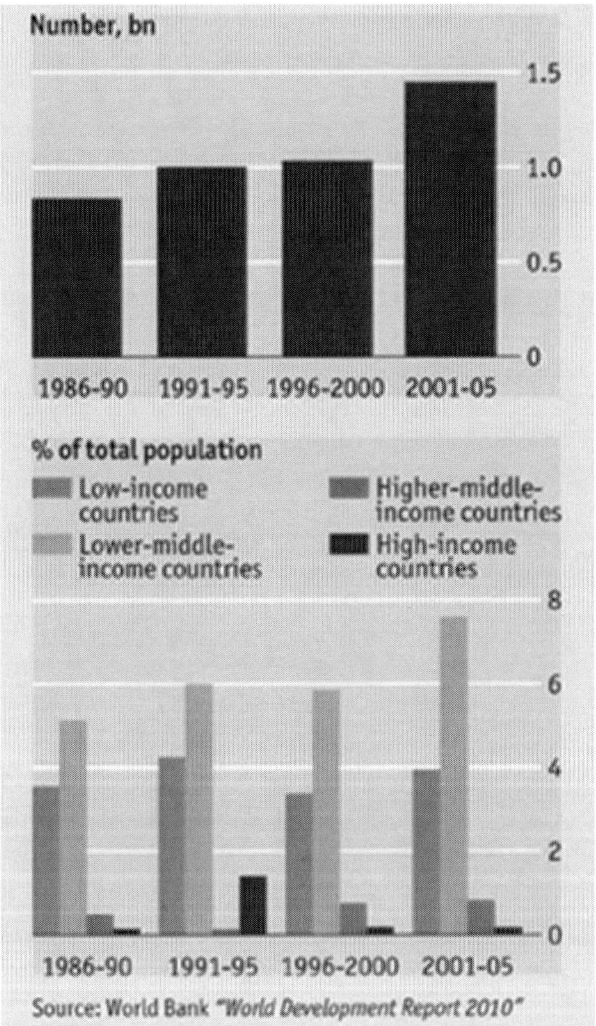

Figure 32. Population affected by climate-related disasters (World Bank "World Development Report 2010").

The potential impact of climate change on health will be more devastating to the developing versus developed countries, simply because there is less access to effective health system infrastructure in the developing countries (Patz et al., 2006). In the U.S. for example, the severity of many chronic diseases was predicted to increase due to climate change (Bernard et al., 2001). The effects of climate change on human health can be characterized as direct and indirect (Maantay and Becker, 2012). Direct and indirect impacts (reduced work performance, reproductive problems, and heart or lung strain) of climate change have significant possibility to increase health care costs and lost workdays (IPCC, 2007; Maantay and Becker, 2012).

Table 22. Categories of climate-change risks to health, according to causal pathway

Risk Category	Causal Pathway
Primary	Direct biologic consequences of heat waves, extreme weather events, and temperature-enhanced levels of urban air pollutants
Secondary	Risks mediated by changes in biophysically and ecologically based processes and systems, particularly food yields, water flows, infectious-disease vectors, and (for zoonotic diseases) intermediate-host ecology
Tertiary	More diffuse effects (e.g., mental health problems in failing farm communities; displaced groups, disadvantaged indigenous and minority ethnic groups) Consequences of tension and conflict owing to climate change-related declines in basic resources (water, food, timber, living space)

Chronic Disease Consequences of Climate Change

This section gives a brief synopsis of what is known about the relationship between climate change and specific diseases. The diseases addressed include cancer, CVD and stroke and diabetes.

Cancer

Cancer is a leading cause of morbidity and mortality worldwide with 8.2 million deaths in 2012. The four most common cancers occurring globally are lung, female breast, bowel and prostate cancer, which account for around 4 in 10 of all cancers diagnosed worldwide (Ferlay et al., 2012). An estimated 14.1 million adults in the world were diagnosed with cancer in 2012 (Figure 33). More than 50% of cancers occur in the developing world. Ferlay et al. (2012) cited lung cancer as the most common cancer in men worldwide (16.7% of all new cases in men; more than one in 10 of all diagnoses, and 10% of deaths. Cancer of the lung cancer caused the most deaths globally, that is, almost 20% of all deaths (Ferlay et al., 2012).

Smoking is the main cause of lung cancer but air pollution, indoor air pollution and fine particulates also contribute to the burden (Beelen et al., 2008; Krewski et al., 2009). Climate change exerts direct and indirect effects on cancer; however, data regarding the mechanism of the linkage between cancer and climate change is linked have not been clearly elucidated. Nonetheless, the climate change/cancer linkage has been associated with exposure to toxic chemicals, and depletion of the stratospheric ozone.

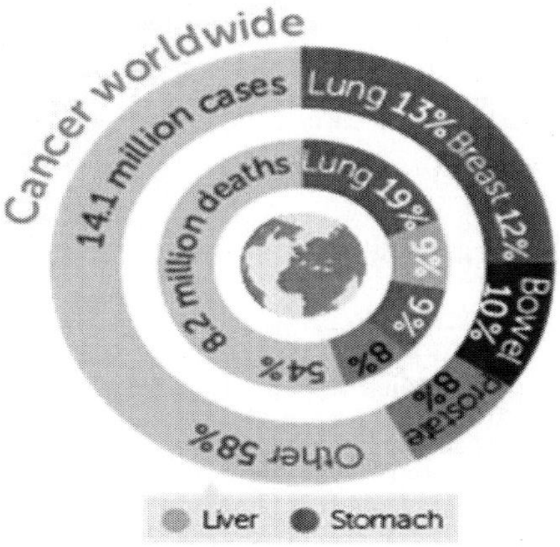

Figure 33. Cancer Worldwide (Ferlay et al., 2012).

Increased Exposure to Toxic Chemicals

One hypothesis put forward for the direct impact of climate change on cancer is through increased exposure to toxic chemicals. Toxic chemicals are known or assumed to be carcinogenic following substantial rainfall, and by escalated volatilization of chemicals under extreme temperature (Portier et al., 2010). To illustrate, heavy rainfall or floods have the potential to increase the leaching of toxic chemicals and heavy metals from storage sites or runoff into water from land containing toxic chemicals, thereby intensifying contamination (Haines et al., 2006). Increases in respiratory diseases have also been reported after flooding in developing and developed countries (Ahern et al., 2005).

Depletion of Stratospheric Ozone

EHP and NIEHS (2010) reported that another direct effect of climate change on health is the depletion of stratospheric ozone, which results in increased ultraviolet (UV) radiation exposure. The stratosphere is the layer of the earth's atmosphere which lies between 10 and 50 km above the earth, and is characterized by little vertical change in temperature (Muir, 1999). The sun is the strongest source of UV radiation in the environment. The UV radiation spectrum is divided into three regions called UVA, UVB and UVC, based on their wavelengths. As sunlight passes through the atmosphere, most of UVC is absorbed by the ozone layer and does not reach the earth's surface. UVC is the most damaging type of UV radiation.

Ozone (O_3) forms naturally in the stratosphere through dissociation of molecular oxygen (O_2) by UV radiation, and subsequent combination of atomic oxygen (O) with O_2 (Muir 1999). UV radiation is short wave, high intensity radiation as shown in the reaction below. The UV radiation that dissociates O_2 is referred to as UVC radiation. It is very short wavelength (<242 nm) and very high intensity radiation.

Reaction

O_2--- $^{(hv)}$-------> O + O

O + O_2 --------> O_3

hv – UV radiation; the reaction takes place in the presence of *hv*

It is known that UV radiation exposure increases the risk of skin cancers. Basal and squamous cell skin cancers are directly correlated to exposure to UV rays. The relationship between skin cancer and climate change is impacted by other factors such as temperature, which can enhance the carcinogenic potential of UV radiation. Rising temperatures have been connected to increases in UV exposure (Muir, 1999). Previous studies have shown that increased UV radiation exposure in combination with certain polycyclic aromatic hydrocarbons (PAHs) can increase the phototoxicity of these compounds and damage DNA (Portier et al., 2010). Increased UV radiation also could impact the human immune system and alter the body's ability to remove the earliest mutant cells that begin the cancer process, although it is unclear whether these changes would be beneficial or detrimental (Portier et al., 2010).

Air pollution has been declared a carcinogen by the World Health Organization because of its strong association with lung cancer (Leber, 2014). There is increasing evidence that air pollution contributes to an unacceptable burden of chronic disease and premature mortality, especially from respiratory and cardiovascular causes (Smith et al., 2009). Respiratory diseases are intensified by warming-induced upsurges in the frequency of ground-level ozone and particulate air pollution (EPA, 2011). Concentrations of ground-level ozone are increasing in most regions (Chen et al., 2004). Troposheric or ground-level ozone is naturally occurring, and is also the main constituent of smog. Ground-level ozone is a secondary pollutant created by chemical reactions between oxides of nitrogen (NOx) and volatile organic compounds (VOCs) in the presence of bright sunlight with high temperatures (Confalonieri et al., 2007). Air pollution has also been linked to an increased risk for bladder cancer.

Cardiovascular Disease and Stroke

Cardiovascular diseases are the single, leading cause of morbidity worldwide (WHO, 2011a). To reiterate, CVDs are a group of disorders of the heart and blood vessels. CVDs include: coronary heart disease, cerebrovascular disease, peripheral arterial disease, rheumatic heart disease, congenital heart disease, deep vein thrombosis and pulmonary embolism. In 2008, approximately 17.3 million people died from CVDs, that is, 30% of all global deaths (WHO, 2011a). The majority of these deaths were from CHD (45% of deaths), stroke (51% of deaths) and hypertension (16.5% of deaths) (WHO, 2011b; Lim et al., 2012; WHO, 2008). More than 80% of CVD deaths occur in developing countries (WHO, 2011a). It is predicted that by 2030, deaths from CVDs will rise to 23.3 million people (WHO, 2011a; Mathers and Loncar, 2006).

CVD is responsible for 10 and 18% of DALYs (healthy years of life lost) lost in developing and developed countries, respectively. Coronary heart disease burden is projected to increase from approximately 47 million DALYs globally in 1990 to 82 million in 2020. Stroke burden is expected to rise from 38 million DALYs globally in 1990 to 61 million in 2020. A proportional increase in cardiovascular disease mortality attributable to climate extremes is projected in tropical regions (Confalonieri et al., 2007).

It has been reported that climate change may aggravate CVD by intensifying heat stress, increasing the body burden of airborne particulates, and modifying the distribution of zoonotic vectors, which trigger infectious diseases linked to CVD (Portier et al., 2010). For example, CVD hospital admissions increased with heat, and dysrhythmias were predominantly associated with extreme cold (Ebi et al., 2004; Schwartz et al., 2004). Cold weather can precipitate heart attacks. Cold spells were associated with positive mean excess CVD mortality in all age groups between 25 and 80+ years, and in both males and females (Kysely et al., 2009). In Kyseley et al.'s 2009 study, the relative mortality effects were most pronounced and direct in middle-aged men (25–59 years).

Ebi et al. (2004) associated increased stroke incidence with rising temperatures. Other less direct pathways of the linkage between climate change and CVD have been cited. The incidence of certain vector-borne and zoonotic diseases (VBZD) has been associated with CVD (Portier et al., 2010). It has been estimated that roughly 10% of strokes in developing countries are related to VBZD, many of which are climate-sensitive (Portier et al., 2010). There is evidence that Chagas disease, an important cause of stroke in many developing countries is climate-sensitive (Carcavallo 1999).

Exposure to elevated concentrations of ozone has been associated with increased hospital admissions for chronic obstructive pulmonary disease, other respiratory diseases and asthma (Bell et al., 2006). In an earlier study conducted by Gong et al., (1998), the researchers concluded that elevated levels of ozone exposure have the capability to increase myocardial work and impair pulmonary gas exchange in persons with preexisting CVD condition. It has been suggested that ozone indirectly exerts cardiovascular effects by impairing alveolar arterial oxygen transfer and potentially reducing O_2 supply to the myocardium, thus creating a need for cardiovascular adjustment (Gong et al., 1998).

Other climate-related exposures have been directly or indirectly linked to the incidence of CVD. For example, the stress of extreme weather occurrences and anxiety over its reappearance has been directly linked to myocardial infarction, sudden cardiac death and cardiomyopathy (Leor et al., 1996; Watanabe et al., 2005; Suzuki et al., 1997). Displacements connected to disasters have been indirectly related to disruptions of medical care, thus placing populations with chronic CVD at risk for disease exacerbation (102 Krausel-Wood et al., 2008 – to get). Generally, the literature pertaining to the direct and indirect effect of climate change on CVD is sparse (Portier et al., 2010). However, it is established that climate change will have a global detrimental effect on the prevalence of CVD (Portier et al., 2010). It is also known that the effect of climate change on CVD from extreme weather events and certain VBZD is also expected to increase in the future (Portier et al., 2010).

Further research into the impact of extreme temperatures, and changes in air quality associated with climate change on CVD is needed. The research findings will provide information to policy makers and populations, which will potentially enhance their decision making ability.

Diabetes

The Linkages

There are direct and indirect linkages between T2D and climate change as shown in Figure 34. Climatic extremes such as drought, disasters and long periods of extreme heat directly increase people's exposure to diabetes risk (Dain and Hadley, 2012). Starvation among pregnant women may even set the scene for type 2 diabetes in their children. During climatic extremities, people with established diabetes suffer adverse health outcomes or are left without access to essential medicines because of destabilized health systems (Dain and Hadley, 2012). The indirect connections between diabetes and climate change refer to the common global forces and trends, such as urbanization, fast-changing demographics, and global food industry practices, which contribute to high-carbon obesogenic environments (Dain and Hadley, 2012).

The explanations for the interconnections are taken from IDF and Bupa (2012). The authors have explained that in terms of the global vectors shown in Figure 34, Type 2 diabetes and climate change have common global vectors including urbanization, changing population demographics, and a globalized food system. The linkage among rapid urbanization, climate change and diabetes is explained. As stated earlier in this book, urbanization can lead to lifestyle change.

People who move to cities increase their chances of developing diabetes through greater exposure to risk factors, such as greater use of motorized transportation, too little physical activity, unhealthy diets and greater exposure to greenhouse gas emissions. The United Kingdom Integrated Panel on climate control indicated that 23% of global GHG emissions are from transport with road traffic contributing 75% of the total emissions (Mackett and Brown, 2011). The demographics increasing size and changing population impact the global food system. The overproduction and consumption of animal products and processed foods high in calories, sugar and saturated fat is increasing diabetes risk and threatens the environment (IDF and Bupa, 2012). The global food trade is the driving force behind the nutrition transition to these foods in low- and middle-income countries.

Figure 34 shows that there are direct connections between type 2 diabetes and climate change. The effects of climate change, including climactic extremes, may increase risk of diabetes in populations by curtailing physical activity, disrupting traditional food supplies, and increasing food insecurity. Extreme climactic events such as heat waves increase morbidity and mortality in people with underlying conditions such as diabetes (McGeekin and Marabelli, 2001).

Individuals with underlying medical conditions such as diabetes are more susceptible to the harmful health impacts of climate change. In warmer climates, dehydration and heatstroke increases morbidity and mortality in people with diabetes. People with diabetes are predisposed to cardiovascular events during heat waves and higher mortality from heart attack on days of high air pollution. Such situations usually damage healthcare infrastructure and their capacity to provide critical care for individuals with diabetes. People with diabetes suffer adverse health outcomes from climatic extremes, for example, diabetes increases vulnerability to dehydration and heat stroke during heat waves (Dain and Hadley, 2012). Disasters such as floods and storms threaten health systems and weaken capacity for diabetes prevention and management. For example, after hurricane Katrina in the U.S. in 2006, vulnerable individuals with chronic diseases such as diabetes were left without access to care and/or medication. It should be noted that developing countries are often faced with the double threat of climatic extremes and high rates of chronic disease.

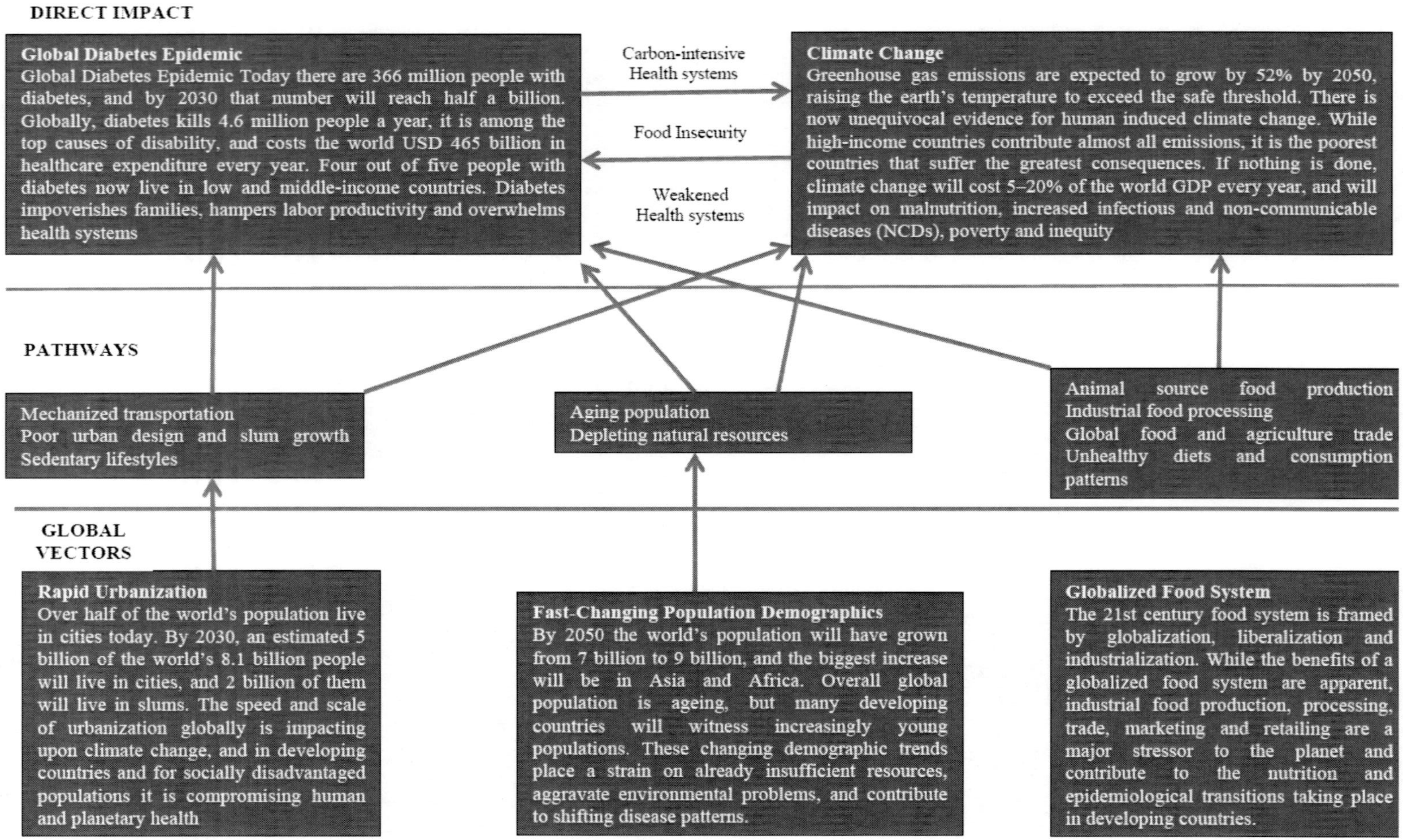

Figure 34. Mapping the interconnections: Type 2 diabetes and climate change (Dain and Hadley, 2012).

According to Edwards and Roberts (2009), there is a linkage between obesity (a major risk factor for diabetes) and greenhouse gas (GHG) from transport and food production. Obese environments usually have larger carbon footprints (WHO and Health Care without Harm, 2009). Increasing obesity prevalence in a population increases GHG emissions from food production and motor vehicle travel. It has been estimated that a population in which 40% of people are obese requires 19% more food energy than a population in which there is a normal BMI distribution (IDF and Bupa, 2012). Climate change is also associated with intensified food insecurity. Climate change usually results in water scarcity and droughts, which in turn impact on food production and supply (IDF and Bupa, 2012). Malnutrition, whether over- or under-nutrition, increases individuals' risk of developing type 2 diabetes and other chronic diseases (IDF and Bupa, 2012).

In sum, the effects of climate change on health are likely to be predominantly negative and impact most heavily on developing countries where the capacity to adapt is weakest. For example, there is less access to effective health system infrastructure in the developing countries. It is predicted that developing countries would bear 80% of the climate change burden. The climate change/cancer linkage has been associated with exposure to toxic chemicals, and depletion of the stratospheric ozone. Increases in respiratory diseases have also been reported after flooding in developing and developed countries. There is increasing evidence that air pollution contributes to an unacceptable burden of chronic disease and premature mortality, especially from respiratory and cardiovascular causes. Climate change may aggravate CVD by intensifying heat stress, increasing the body burden of airborne particulates, and modifying the distribution of zoonotic vectors, which trigger infectious diseases linked to CVD. For example, CVD hospital admissions increased with heat, and dysrhythmias were predominantly associated with extreme cold. Disasters such as floods and storms could further threaten the fragile health systems in developing countries, and weaken capacity for diabetes prevention and management. Mitigation policies should be put into place to reduce the effects of climate change on chronic disease in developing countries. Governments should ensure that populations better understand the relationship between climate change and chronic disease for improved prevention and management of chronic diseases.

Part IV: Summing up

Chapter 8

Case Studies; Evidence-Based Interventions

This chapter highlights a number of studies and evidence-based interventions, which have been reported in the literature.

Case 1

Chronic Non-Communicable Diseases in Cameroon - Burden, Determinants and Current Policies (Echouffo-Tcheugui and Kengne, 2011)

Cameroon

Cameroon is located in the western part of the Central African region. It is bordered by the Republic of Congo, Gabon and Equatorial Guinea to its south, Central African Republic to its east, Chad to its northeast, Gulf of Guinea to the southwest and Nigeria in the west (Figure 35). It is nearly twice the size of Oregon or slightly larger than California. It has an area of 475,440 sq. km and is classified as a lower-middle-income country (Table 1) with a gross GNI of US$1,046-$4,125. Its GDP per capita is $1,167 and a real GDP growth rate of 4.7% (Table 1). The World Bank estimates from 2014 indicate a population of roughly 23,130,708. According to WHO statistics, roughly, 57.6% individuals live in urban areas, a population that grew at a rate of 3.90% annually from 2005 to 2010.

Echouffo-Tcheugui and Kengne (2011) concluded that Cameroon may now be experiencing the double burden of infectious and chronic diseases. Chronic diseases in Cameroon accounted for an estimated 31% of all mortality (239,000) in 2008. The most prevalent NCDs in Cameroon are cardiovascular diseases, which accounted for 14% of total deaths across all age groups in 2008. In 2008, non-communicable variants of respiratory diseases, cancers and diabetes contributed 4, 3 and 2%, respectively, to total mortality (Commonwealth Health Online, 2015). In 2002, chronic diseases including CVD, diabetes, cancers and respiratory diseases accounted for 848.1 deaths per 100,000, that is, 1,480 DALYs per 1,000 and 21% of total DALYs (Echouffo-Tcheugui and Kengne, 2011).

According to the WHO (2014b), in Cameroon, the probability of dying between the ages of 30 and 70 years from the four main chronic diseases is 20%.

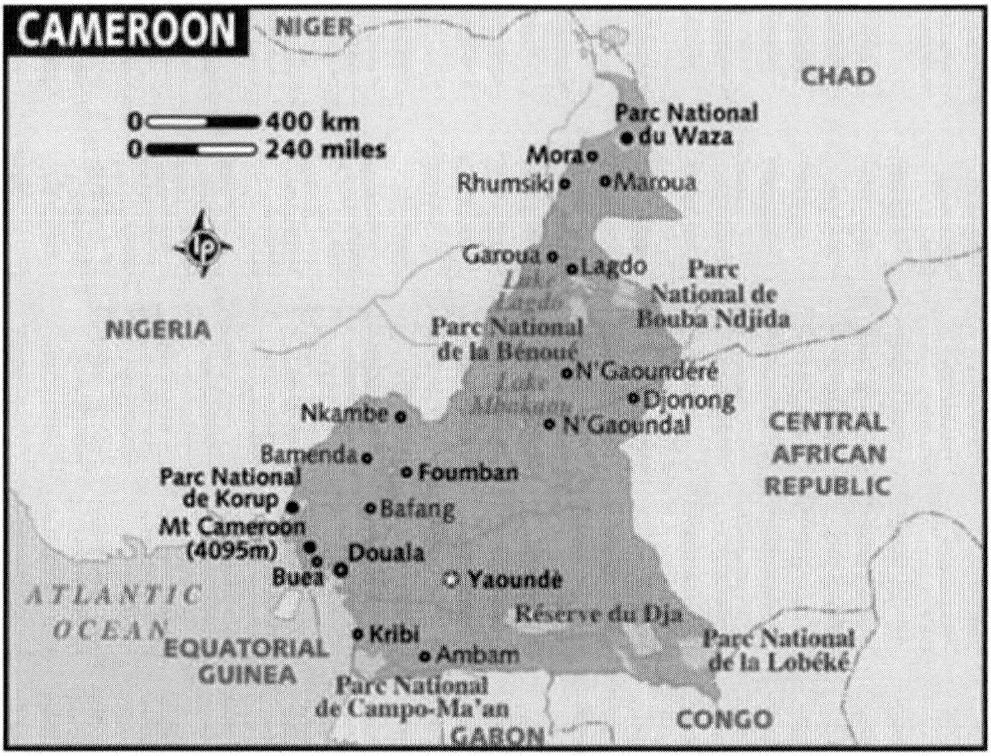

Figure 35. Map of Cameroon (http://www.lonelyplanet.com/maps/africa/cameroon).

Over a 10-year period (1994-2003) there was an almost 10-fold increase in diabetes prevalence in Cameroonian adults (Mbanya et al., 2006; Assah and Mbanya, 2009). In 2010, the IDF estimated the national prevalence of diabetes among adults aged 20 to 79 years at 4.4%. The prevalence of undiagnosed diabetes was roughly 80% (Mbanya et al., 2006). The most current IDF estimate for diabetes in Cameroon is shown in Table 23. Assah and Mbanya (2009) reported that glycemic control in known diabetes patients was often very poor with only about one in four known diabetic patients in a population-based survey had optimal fasting blood glucose levels.

It has been speculated that the prevalence of physical inactivity in Cameroon is increasing, especially in urban areas (Assah et al., 2011; Assah et al., 2009; Sobngwi et al., 2002). However, studies providing population-based or nation-wide data on levels of physical activity or sedentary time are lacking. Assah et al. (2009) concluded that physical activity energy expenditure (PAEE) is inversely associated with 2-h glucose independently of adiposity or fitness. The authors suggested that interventions aimed at increasing PAEE could play an important role in diabetes and CVD prevention in developing countries.

In terms of response to chronic diseases, Cameroon has no: i) evidence-based national guidelines/protocols/standards for the management of major NCDs through a primary care approach; ii) NCD surveillance and monitoring system in place to enable reporting against the nine global NCD targets; iii) national, population-based cancer registry; iv) operationalized

NCD unit/branch within the Ministry of Health or equivalent; and v) operational multi-sectorial national policy or action plan, which integrates several NCDs and shared risk factors (WHO, 2014b). Cameroon needs an integrated approach to health care, which accounts for chronic diseases if it is to curb the rise that is being experienced. Additionally, guidelines for the management of chronic diseases, surveillance and monitoring system and a national policy which integrates the most common chronic diseases need to be put into place.

Table 23. International Diabetes Federation summary estimates for Cameroon and Jamaica, 2014

Country	Diabetes cases (20-79) in 1000s	Undiagnosed diabetes cases (20-79) in 1000s	Diabetes national prevalence (%)	Diabetes comparative prevalence (%)	Diabetes-related deaths (20-79)	Cost/person with diabetes* (USD)
Cameroon	24.51	18.40	6.9	8.38	13,821.95	108.87
Jamaica	182.82	45.96	10.76	10.53	1,828.49	460.98

Case 2

Profile of Cardiac Diagnosis in Cameroon and Impact on Healthcare Services (Tchoumi and Butera, 2013)

The prevalence of chronic disease and in particular CVD is increasing in the Cameroon. CVD is a major public health problem in the Cameroon, which is burdensome to the healthcare system (Tchoumi and Butera, 2013). *The country has 178 health districts, with 162 districts hospitals among which only 154 are operational. Additionally, Cameroon has 2,043 public medical structures, mainly concentrated in urban zones. As is typical in developing countries, Cameroon extensively used public resources to support health system, but the declining GDP, among other things has resulted in reduced resources to the health system. For example, Cameroon has 1,555 physicians, that is, one doctor per 12,500 persons, which is among one of the lowest in the world (Tchoumi and Butera, 2013). According to Tchoumi and Butera (2013), the causes for the shortages of health workers including factors such as brain drain to the private sector and other countries, low salaries, poor working conditions and insufficient training capacities. Within the health system, family members cover for the cost of treatments, which is usually unaffordable, which usually leads to non-compliance and adherence. Furthermore, paying for health care often competes with financial commitments for other things such as children's education and food* (Tchoumi and Butera, 2013). Out-of-pocket payments for treatment are required to sustain the healthcare system. Between 2008 and 2009 Cameroonian households were paying 77 to 90% of the annual total health expenditures (Egbe, 2013). These out-of-pocket payments impact negatively on healthcare accessibility and have the tendency to increase inequities in accessing healthcare.

Tchoumi and Butera (2013) investigated the preparedness of health care services for 8,389 adult patients and 706 children presenting with CVD in St. Elizabeth catholic general hospital Shisong, Cardiac Center. In their findings, Tchoumi and Butera (2013) diagnosed

29.6 and 41.5% of the patients with CHF and hypertension, respectively (Figure 36). Between 1994 and 1998, the prevalence rates for hypertension and diabetes doubled for urban Cameroonian males (1994 – 8.3 and 1.1%; 1998 – 17.6 and 6.2% for hypertension and diabetes, respectively). Tchoumi and Butera (2013) reported 46.5% hypertension prevalence for 2010 in a rural center. Hypertension was associated with diabetes in 11% cases.

Out-of-pocket payments for treatment are required to sustain the healthcare system in Cameroon. The catastrophic effect of out-of-pocket payments on families has been discussed throughout the book. Healthcare systems in developing countries must be improved if the halt in chronic disease is to be realized.

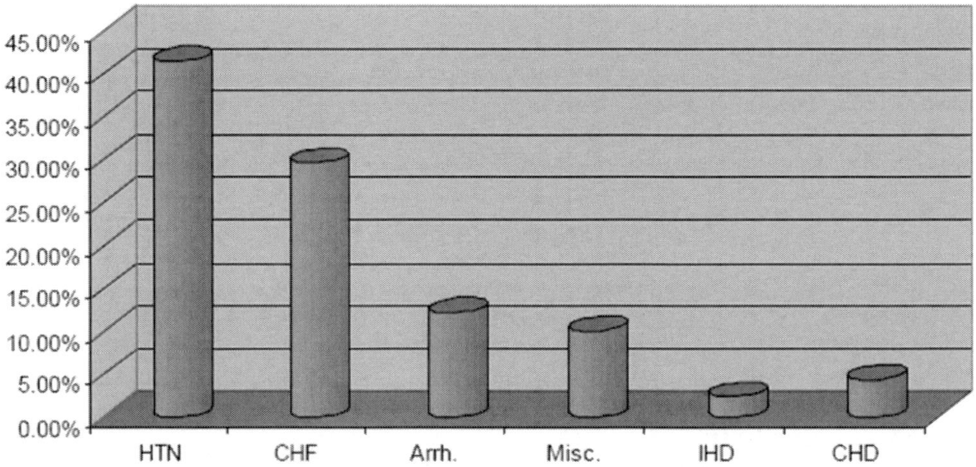

Figure 36. Cardiovascular diseases represented in the Cardiac Center of St. Elizabeth Catholic General hospital. Notes: HTN - Hypertension; CHF - Congestive heart failure; Arrh. - Arrhythmia; Misc. - Miscellaneous; IHD - Ischemic heart disease; CHD - Congenital heart disease (Tchoumi and Butera, 2013).

Case 3

Project Title: Agita São Paulo (Arogya World, 2011)

Purpose of the Case Study: To highlight how Agita São Paulo has been able to get millions of Brazilians in the state of São Paulo to increase their physical activity level and transform the behavior of entire communities.

Objectives: Agita São Paulo has two objectives, namely to: i) increase the public's knowledge of the importance of physical activity; and ii) increase the levels of physical activity among the citizens of São Paulo. Additionally, they sought to establish partnerships with governmental and NGOs to ensure the program's success.

Approach: Brazil is an upper middle-income developing country with a high prevalence of chronic disease. Roughly 88% of people aged 40 years and over suffers from one chronic disease while 26% suffer from at least three chronic diseases (Carvalho et al., 2012). The Agita São Paulo initiative was launched in 1996 as a response to the escalating level of physical inactivity in Brazil, and increasing mortality from chronic disease, especially within the state of São Paulo. Agita means to move the body, or to move the crowd; it also represents changing ways of thinking and becoming more active (Matsudo et al., 2003). Agita São Paulo has been characterized as a model for other developing countries by WHO (Matsudo et al., 2003).

Fundamentally, the program encourages people to adopt an active lifestyle by amassing at least 30 minutes of moderate physical activity daily on most days of the week (Matsudo et al., 2003). The initiative targets three specific groups, students, workers, and the elderly. Large numbers of individuals are reached through mega events conducted with partner organizations and networks that help take the program message deep into communities. These mega events usually take place in major cities or involve at least one million citizens. For example, 'Agita Galera' is held annually in partnership with the Department of Education. On the last Friday of August, 6,000 public schools in the state of São Paulo are mobilized, regular classes are replaced by Agita classes, and 7 to 18 year-old students participate in walks, sports and other creative activities that increase students' levels of physical activity as well as their awareness of the benefits. Private schools, which do not participate in Agita Galera have 33% less physical activity levels than the public schools (AROGYA World, 2011; Matsudo et al., 2003).

Additionally, since the Agita São Paulo initiative began, it has been able to greatly increase the levels of physical activity among the citizens of São Paulo, as measured by multiple surveys and studies. A few more examples of results obtained:

- One group of elderly women reported that their physical activity was increased from 3.5 to 5 days per week, and from 40 to 120 minutes per day (Matsudo et al., 2003).
- In one school the initiative led to an increased number of students obtaining the proper amount of exercise each week, with the level for males rising from 20% to 40% and the level for females rising form 4% to 42% (Matsudo et al., 2003).
- A health insurance company applied the Agita method and realized an increase in physical activity among diabetes and hypertension patients from 23% to 53% (Matsudo et al., 2003)

Key to Success

- Simple messages
- Effective marketing
- Focus on moderate as opposed to vigorous activity
- By framing the daily physical activity requirements as moderate activities that can be accumulated in small portions throughout the day, people believed that physical activity goals were achievable and more manageable. For example, 10 minutes of activity three times per day met the daily requirement of 30 minutes per day
- Cost-effective large scale public health intervention for chronic disease prevention

Agita São Paulo is a simple cost-effective initiative, which has greatly increased the levels of physical activity among the citizens of São Paulo. This is a simple strategy that could be adopted by developing countries with collaborations and partnerships, regardless of resource levels.

Case 4

Program Title: mDiabetes (arogyaworld.org)

Objective

To reach more than one million people from all over India with text messages in 12 languages about diabetes and its prevention, and to measure the program's effectiveness in bringing about behavior change known to prevent diabetes.

Approach

mDiabetes was designed and implemented by Arogya World in collaboration with Nokia Life, Emory University, Johnson & Johnson, Aetna, Biocon and Ipsos. Sixty-plus million Indians live with diabetes and one million die from it annually. Indians get the disease an average of 10 years earlier than counterparts in the West, often in their third and fourth decades. Untreated, diabetes can lead to complications such as heart disease, blindness, amputations and kidney failure. Mobile phones are widely used in India, throughout different geographic regions and socio-economic backgrounds. There are said to be about 900 million cell phone subscribers in India. Importantly, the WHO emphasizes that approximately 80% of heart disease and diabetes, and 40% of cancers can be prevented through healthy lifestyles such as avoiding tobacco use, eating healthy foods and increasing daily physical activity.

mDiabetes has been designed as a population-level nationwide public health intervention using mobile technology to establish health behaviors known to prevent diabetes. In 2012, Nokia Life helped Arogya World recruit 1,052,633 persons who opted-in to receive mDiabetes text messages. Messages were provided free to the consumers twice a week for six months. Participants came from all over India and a variety of socio-economic backgrounds. Fifty six text messages were designed based on science and behavior change theory, and then consumer-tested in simulated and real world conditions. The messages were refined, and then culturally adapted for Indian audiences based on consumer feedback and review. More than 56 million mDiabetes text messages were transmitted to the consumers throughout 2012.

Effectiveness

Program effectiveness was assessed by comparing responses of 950 consumers, based on telephone interviews, before and after they received the messages, and also by comparing them with the responses of a similar number of consumers who did not receive mDiabetes messages. Preliminary results indicate that consumers' awareness of diabetes and its complications increased.

Promising trends in behavior change were noted:

- An 11% increase in daily exercise
- A 15% increase in the intake of 2-3 servings of fruits a day
- An 8% increase in 2-3 servings of vegetables a day

Next Steps

Once effectiveness is fully established, scale-up of the program to reach and help millions more in India is a planned next step. Expansion geographically to other countries, in partnership with global health organizations, governments and private sector partners, is a possibility. mDiabetes has the potential to become a core part of the chronic disease prevention model for the developing world.

Case 5

The Chronic Disease Dilemma in the Caribbean Region and Jamaica

Hospedales et al. (2011) and Hennis et al. (2004) reported that the English-speaking Caribbean region has the highest death rates due to chronic diseases in the Americas. Augustine (2007), Eldemire-Shearer et al. (2011), Pan American Health Organization/ Caribbean Community (2006) indicating that NCDs such as diabetes, HD and stroke are the main causes of mortality in the Caribbean. In the region of the Americas, 30.0% of all deaths are caused by preventable NCDs that occur prematurely (<70 years) (Mathers et al., 2001). The English-speaking Caribbean countries with a population of 7.5 million are the worst affected by the chronic disease epidemic in the Americas. According to (Hennis et al., 2004) diabetes-related lower extremity amputations in Barbados are among the highest recorded in the world ((Hennis et al., 2004). Comparing Trinidad and Tobago with North America, diabetes mortality is six times higher, CVD is 84% higher and cervical cancer rates are three to 12 times higher (PAHO, 2009). In the last five decades, hypertension, diabetes, and CVD have grown exponentially.

Jamaica, a country in the English-speaking Caribbean region, experienced an increase in chronic diseases over the last 10 years (Bourne et al., 2014a; Bourne et al., 2010; Bourne and Charles, 2011; Bourne, 2012; Bourne, 2013; Wilks et al., 2013). The rate of chronic diseases in Jamaica increased from eight to 56 per 1,000 in 2002 and 2007, respectively (Bourne et al., 2010). The detailed increase in diabetes was 185%, hypertension, 12.7%, and five in every 100 individuals with diabetes were less than 30 years of age (Bourne et al. 2014b). Jamaican mortality statistics have revealed that CVD, cancers, HD, diabetes, and hypertension are among the top ten leading causes of death (Bourne et al., 2014b). The high prevalence of chronic disease seen in Jamaica mirrors the pattern across the Caribbean (Hospedales et al., 2011; Mathers et al., 2009; James et al., 2010). The most current IDF estimate for diabetes in Jamaica shows a national prevalence of 10.76% (Table 23).

Wilks et al. (2008) conducted a cross-sectional probability survey of 2,848 Jamaicans ages 15-74 years. Their findings indicated that 51.7, 7.9, 25.2, 35.3 and 11.7% of the individuals were overweight or obese; diabetic; hypertensive; pre-hypertensive and had high cholesterol, respectively. According to the researchers, about half of those with hypertension, 76.1% of the diabetics and 14.0% of those with raised cholesterol were unaware of their condition. Compared with the British Virgin Islands, the prevalence of hypertension and diabetes in Jamaica is higher. The numbers for the British Virgin Islands are 16.6 and 10.0% for hypertension and diabetes, respectively. However, the burden of chronic disease in Jamaica is similar to that in the Cameroon, British Virgin Islands, South Africa and the rest of the world (James et al., 2010; Echouffo-Tcheugui and Kengne, 2011; Mayosi et al., 2009; WHO, 2011a).

Response to Chronic Diseases in the Caribbean

The history of the Caribbean community (CARICOM) collaboration in the prevention and control of chronic disease dates back to 1986. In 1986, the Caribbean Cooperation in Health initiative approved by Ministers of Health included chronic diseases as a priority area. The 2001 CARICOM Heads of Government Nassau Declaration, "The Wealth of the Region" gave direction to a regional approach to chronic diseases. The Caribbean Commission on Health and Development, 2005 named NCDs a super priority. In 2007, the CARICOM Heads of Government Summit on NCDs issued the 15-point NCD Summit Declaration, "Uniting to Stop the Epidemic of Chronic NCDs." The Summit focused on prevention and control of NCDs and gave clear policy directions for an inter-sectorial approach that addresses many key risk factors.

In the Caribbean, alcohol abuse has not been adequately addressed, and the health sector has not made sufficient progress in implementing evidence-based preventive treatment for people living with NCDs, despite the regional political and institutional commitment (Hospedales et al., 2011). Bourne et al. (2014b) argued that there has been a steady increase in chronic diseases in Jamaica and the implemented programs aimed at decreasing the prevalence have been ineffective. Supporting evidence for their arguments from the Summit of the Heads of Government of the Caribbean Community on NCDs in the Caribbean, Port of Spain, Trinidad in 2007, which gave clear policy directives to address the rising NCDs epidemic in the Caribbean region (CARICOM Secretariat, 2007). However, outcomes were far from effective. Overall, inadequate funding and lack of ownership have negatively impacted the implementation of these initiatives (Hospedales et al., 2011).

Chapter 9

Taking Action

The Direction and Way Forward

Global Goals

Urgent actions are needed to halt the escalating prevalence of chronic diseases in developing countries and the rest of the world. In 2011, the United Nations (UN) held the High-level Meeting (HLM) on the Prevention and Control of NCDs. This was historic in that it was only the second time that the UN General Assembly convened to discuss a specific health issue. The HLM led to greater global attention to NCDs and called for new global targets and an action plan for addressing NCDs. Among the targets subsequently outlined in the *WHO Global Action Plan for the Prevention and Control of NCDs, 2013–2020* (WHO, 2013) are:

- A 25% relative reduction in risk of premature mortality from cardiovascular diseases, cancer, diabetes, or chronic respiratory diseases
- At least 10% relative reduction in the harmful use of alcohol, as appropriate, within the national context
- A 10% relative reduction in prevalence of insufficient physical activity
- A 30% relative reduction in mean population intake of salt/sodium
- A 30% relative reduction in prevalence of current tobacco use in persons aged 15-plus years
- 25% relative reductions in the prevalence of raised blood pressure or contain the prevalence of raised blood pressure, according to national circumstances
- Halt the rise in diabetes and obesity
- At least 50% of eligible people receive drug therapy and counseling (including glycemic control) to prevent heart attacks and strokes
- An 80% availability of the affordable basic technologies and essential medicines, including generics, required to treat major NCDs in both public and private facilities (WHO, 2013).

Selected Responses to the Targets

In 2013, the World Health Organization adopted the non-communicable Disease (NCD) Monitoring Framework, which monitors nine voluntary global targets for 2025. Outcomes from the global target to "halt the rise in diabetes and obesity" were unimpressive. Only Djibouti, Iceland, Malta, Nauru and Venezuela have halted the rise of the diabetes indicator (raised blood glucose) (IFPRI, 2015).

Country progress in controlling diabetes rates further revealed that 185 countries had increased rates or were "off course," and 13 countries have shown a halt in rate among women (IFPRI, 2015).

Interventions

Several simple, evidence-based and/or cost-effective interventions for addressing chronic diseases have been demonstrated across the globe. Table 24 shows a sample intervention plan for prevention/control of diabetes and hypertension in different health care settings. To summarize these interventions:

Prevention

- Interventions, which target modifiable risk factors and promote healthy living, such as: i) education and awareness about chronic diseases and their risk factors; ii) efforts to prevent and reduce the use of tobacco and the harmful use of alcohol; and iii) creating environments, which support increased consumption of fruit and vegetables, reduced salt intake, and increased physical activity.

Management

- Measures to support effective treatment and quality care (with particular attention to the needs of the poor and most vulnerable, including those with major chronic diseases). This includes building the capacity of health systems and health workers to respond effectively to chronic diseases, and making basic medicines and technologies needed to manage chronic disease available and accessible.

Advocacy

- Efforts to raise the priority accorded to chronic disease at the global and national levels;
- Integration of chronic disease prevention and control into governments and multilateral institutions' policies, plans, and programs, and to promote legislative, regulatory, and fiscal measures, which support healthy eating and physical activity and discourages the use of tobacco and alcohol.
- A more holistic approach through collaborations (public health, education, business, and other stakeholders) to prevent and control chronic disease (Mohan et al., 2013)

Table 24. Sample action plans for prevention/control of diabetes and hypertension in different health care settings (Mohan et al., 2013)

	Detection	Diabetes education	Equipment	Medicines
Primary	Large scale screening using high risk category approach	Through community Workers, training of community workers in screening activities	Basic equipment like Glucometer, blood pressure apparatus	Essential low cost generic drugs to be made available at all PHCs
Secondary	Confirmation of diagnosis Screening for complications of diabetes and co-morbid conditions	(i) Physicians (ii) Paramedicals	Ophthalmology Basic laboratory support	Insulin, oral hypoglycemic drugs, ACE inhibitors, calcium antagonists, ARBs, statins, aspirin, and other antihypertensive drugs
Tertiary	Treatment of complications	(i) Diabetologists (ii) Ophthalmologists (iii) Nephrologists (iv) Cardiologists	Advanced equipment (i) Laser photocoagulation (ii) Fundus camera (iii) Cardiac care (iv) Dialysis unit (v) Transplantation	All of above and costlier drugs or treatments

Conclusion

In general, healthcare systems in developing countries are fragile and should be strengthened for effective prevention and control of chronic diseases. Strategies to prevent and control chronic diseases should be population-based, incorporating multilevel, multicomponent, and socio-environmental approaches and integrating community resources with public health and clinical care (Mohan et al., 2013). According to the chronic care model (Figure 18), six areas need improvement to facilitate chronic care in developing countries: community resources; health systems; self-management support; decision support; delivery system redesign; and clinical information systems. These areas highlight the need for policy changes and greater community involvement as shown in the Innovate Care for Chronic conditions Framework (Figure 19).

Throughout the book, various interventions/strategies have been described, which could improve health care for chronic disease, some are shown in Figure 37 taken from Mohan et al. (2013). Although some progress has been made, developing countries are still facing an escalating burden from chronic diseases, which is impacting negatively on sustainable development. Developing countries urgently need to scale up chronic disease prevention and control programs to circumvent this escalating dilemma. The role of governments in developing countries is critical to the development and implementation of well-informed risk-factor chronic disease prevention and control programs. Reallocation of healthcare budgets, policy and system changes, partnerships with NGOs and food industry are essential to reduce chronic disease risk in populations.

Populations in developing countries need to be more aware about basic prevention measures. Governments, private entities, stakeholders, health professionals, civil societies, all must support chronic disease prevention/control by legislation, building human resource capacity for healthcare workers, public education to reduce dietary fat, salt and sugar, food pricing policies, tobacco control, food formulation and changes as discussed to healthcare delivery systems. Chronic disease prevention/control needs to be placed higher on the political agenda of developing countries, policy makers should be fully informed with the up-to-date evidence about the burden and far reaching impacts of chronic diseases. Governments must support the effort with the necessary resources and firm commitment. Private entities, community members, individuals, families and family members must join in the coordinated and focused effort to halt the escalating dilemma of chronic diseases in developing countries.

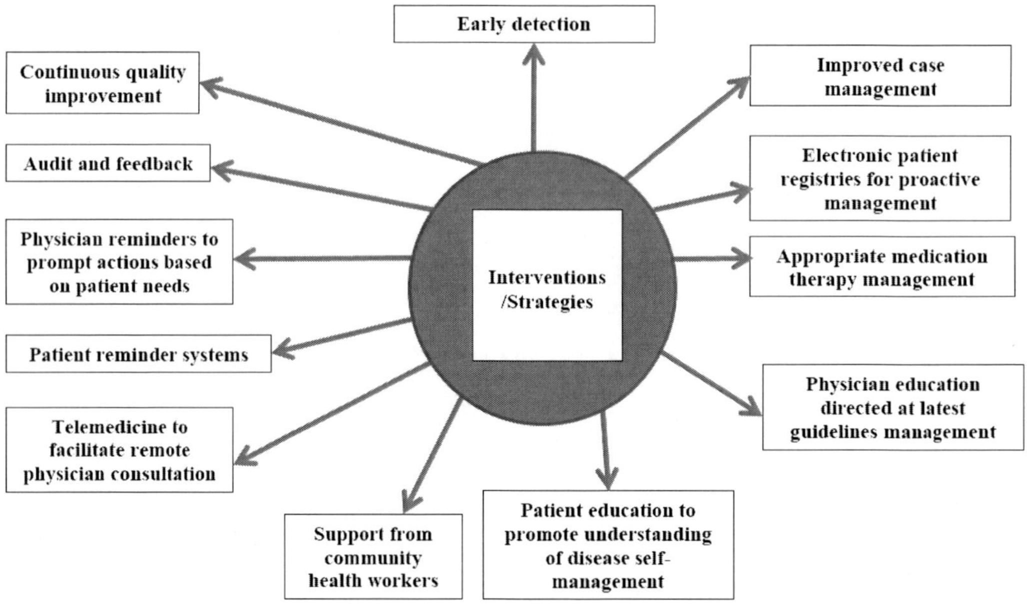

Figure 37. Interventions/Strategies to improve healthcare for chronic disease (Mohan et al., 2013)

Looking Ahead

Chronic diseases will continue to rise and hamper economic and developmental growth in lower and middle income countries if serious action is not taken to address the key risk factors and determinants. There is a need for governments to prioritize funding for healthcare. Looking ahead, the biggest challenge faced by governments in developing countries is the problem of the double burden of disease (infectious and chronic) and the realignment of the healthcare system to facilitate chronic disease prevention and control. Serious decisions will have to be made in a timely fashion to avert the escalating dilemma chronic diseases pose to the developing world.

References

Abbato S. 2008. A Healthier Gold Coast: The role of Non-Government Organizations.

Abdel-Wahab, M., Bourque J-M, Pynda Y., Izewska J., Van der Merwe D., Zubizarreta E., Rosenblatt E. 2013. Status of radiotherapy resources in Africa: an international Atomic Energy Agency analysis. *Lancet Oncology* 14:e168-e175.

Abdulganiyu G., Fola T. 2014. What is the cost of illness of type II diabetes mellitus in a developing economy? *Internat J Pharm Pharm Sci* 6 (Suppl 2):927-931.

Abrahams Z, Mchiza Z, Steyn NP. 2011. Diet and mortality rates in Sub-Saharan Africa: stages in the nutrition transition. *BMC Public Health* 11:801.

ACS (American Cancer Society). 2014. Cancer facts and figures 2014. Atlanta, GA, ACS.

Afroz A. 2012. Economic burden of Type 2 diabetes mellitus: Direct cost, indirect cost and nutritional cost of Type 2 diabetes mellitus in a selected Bangladeshi population, ISBN-10: 3659153044, LAP LAMBERT Academic Publishing.

Aguiree F., Brown A., Cho N., Ho D., Gisela D., Dunning S., Hirst T., Hwang M., Magliano C. et al. 2013. IDF Diabetes Atlas: sixth edition, 6th ed., International Diabetes Federation, Basel, Switzerland.

Ahern M., Kovats RS, Wilkinson P., Few R., Matthies F. 2005. Global health impacts of floods: Epidemiologic evidence. *Epidemiol Rev* 27:36-46.

Albala C, Vio F, Kain J, Uauy R. 2001. Nutrition transition in Latin America: the case of Chile. *Nutr Rev* 59:170-176.

Allender S, Wickramasinghe K, Goldacre M, Matthews D, Katulanda P. 2011. Quantifying urbanization as a risk factor for non communicable disease. *J Urban Health* 88:906–918.

Allender S., Lacey B., Webster P., Rayner M., Deepa M., Scarborough P., et al. 2010. Level of urbanization and non-communicable disease risk factors in Tamil Nadu, India. *Bull World Health Org* 88:297-304.

Alhowaish AK. 2013. Economic costs of diabetes in Saudi Arabia. *J Fam Comm Med* 20:1–7.

Al-Maskari F. 2010. Lifestyle diseases: An economic burden on the health services. UN Chronicle XLVII 2 2010.

Anand K., Shah B., Yadav K., Singh R., Mathur P., Paul E., Kapoor SK. 2007. Are the urban poor vulnerable to non-communicable diseases? A survey of risk factors for non-communicable diseases in urban slums of Faridabad. *Med J India* 20:115–120.

Angkurawaranon C., Jiraporncharoen W., Chenthanakij B., Doyle P., Nitsch D. 2014. Urbanization and non-communicable disease in Southeast Asia: a review of current evidence. Pub Health http://dx.doi.org/10.1016/j.puhe.2014.08.003

Anon. 2013. Mexico passes 'junk food tax' reform. BBC News Online 1/11/2013. Available at: http://www.bbc.co.uk/news/world-latin-america-24766027; accessed 01/10/2014.

AROGYA World. 2011. A case study on Agita São Paulo: Defeating non-communicable diseases through physical activity. Changing the course of chronic disease. Case study 1. Available at: www.arogyaworld.org; accessed 09/22/2015.

Assah FK, Mbanya JC. 2009. Diabetes in sub-Saharan Africa - overview of a looming health challenge. *European Endocrinology* 5:13–17.

Assah FK, Ekelund U, Brage S, Mbanya JC, Wareham NJ. 2011. Urbanization, physical activity, and metabolic health in sub-saharan Africa. *Diabetes Care* 34:491–496.

Assah FK, Ekelund U, Brage S, Mbanya JC, Wareham NJ. 2009. Free-living physical activity energy expenditure is strongly related to glucose intolerance in Cameroonian adults independently of obesity. *Diabetes Care* 32:367–369.

Augustine S. 2007. Facing the challenge of the CNCD epidemic: The global situation and Caribbean perspective. WHO.

Avezum A Braga J, Santos I, Guimaraes HP et al. 2009. Cardiovascular disease in South America: current status and opportunities for prevention. *Heart* (British Cardiac Society) 95:1475–1482.

Balbus JM, Malina C. 2009. Identifying vulnerable subpopulations for climate change health effects in the United States. *Internat J Occup Environ Med* 51:27-33.

Barr VJ, Robinson S, Marin-Link B, Underhill L, Dotts A, Ravensdale D, Salivaras S. 2011. The expanded Chronic Care Model: an integration of concepts and strategies from population health promotion and the Chronic Care Model. *Hosp Q* 7:73–82.

Barcelo A., Aedo C., Rajpathak S., Robles S. 2003. The cost of diabetes in Latin America and the Caribbean. *Bull WHO* 81:19-27.

Barrio-Lopez MT, Martinez-Gonzalez MA, Fernandez-Montero A, Beunza JJ, Zazpe I, Bes-Rastrollo M. 2013. Prospective study of changes in sugar-sweetened beverage consumption and the incidence of the metabolic syndrome and its components: the SUN cohort. *Br J Nutr* 110:1722–31.

Barquera S, Hernández-Barrera L., Campos-Nonato I., Espinosa J., Flores M., Barriguete JA, Rivera JA. 2009. Energy and nutrient consumption in adults: analysis of the Mexican national health and nutrition survey 2006. *Salud Publica Mex* 51:S562–S573.

Barquera S, Campos I, Rivera JA. 2014. Mexico attempts to tackle obesity: the process, results, push-backs, and future challenges. *Obes Rev* 14:69-78.

Basu S, Yoffe P, Hills N, Lustig RH. 2013a. The relationship of sugar to population-level diabetes prevalence: an economic analysis of repeated cross-sectional data. *PLoS ONE,* 8: e57873. doi:10.1371/journal.pone.0057873.

Basu S, Stuckler D, McKee M, Galea G. 2013b. Nutritional determinants of worldwide diabetes: an econometric study of food markets and diabetes prevalence in 173 countries. *Public Health Nutr* 16:179–186.

Batra, R. et al. 2009. Effects of brand local and nonlocal origin on consumer attitudes in developing countries. *J Consumer Psychol* 9:83-95.

Beelen R., Hoek G., van den Brandt PA, Goldbohm RA, Fischer P., Schouten LJ, Armstrong B., Brunekreef B. 2008. Long-term exposure to traffic-related air pollution and lung cancer risk. *Epidemiology* 19:702–710.

Bell ML, Peng RD, Dominici F. 2006. The exposure-response curve for ozone and risk of mortality and the adequacy of current ozone regulations. *Environ Health Persp* 114:532-536.

Berardi N., Sevestre P., Tepaut M., Vigneron A. 2012. The impact of a "soda tax" on prices. Evidence from French microdata. Document De Travail No. 415. Available at: http://www.banque-france.fr; accessed 09/21/2015.

Beran D. et al. 2008. Report on the Rapid Assessment Protocol for Insulin Access in Vietnam (London: International Insulin Foundation, 2008). Available at: http://www.access2insulin.org; accessed 7/13/2015.

Bernard SM, Samet JM, Grambsch A., Ebi KL, Romieu I. 2001. The potential impacts of climate variability and change on air pollution-related health effects in the United States. *Environ Health Persp* 109:(Suppl 2) 199-209.

Bhuyan KK. 2004. Health promotion through self-care and community participation: Elements of a proposed programme in the developing countries. *BMC Public Health* 4:11.

Bibbins-Domingo K, Chertow GM, Coxson PG, Moran A, Lightwood JM, Pletcher MJ, et al. 2010. Projected effect of dietary salt reductions on future cardiovascular disease. *N Engl J Med* 362:590-9.

Black, R.E. 1990. Prevention in developing countries. *J General Internal Medicine* 5 (5 Suppl):132-135.

Blair SN, Brodney S. 1999. Effects of physical activity and obesity on morbidity and mortality: Current evidence and research issues. *Med Sci Sports Exerc* 31:S646-662. Bloom DE, Cafiero ET, Jane-Llopis E., Abrahams-Gessel S., Bloom LR, Fathima S, Feigl AB, Gaziano T., Mowafi M., Pandya A., Prettner K., Rosenberg L., Seligman B., Stein AZ, Weinstein C.. 2011. The global economic burden of non-communicable diseases. Geneva: World Economic Forum. Available at: www.weforum.org/EconomicsOfNCD.

Bloomberg Philanthropies. 2013. Supporting strong policies to reduce rising rates of obesity. Available at: http://www.bloomberg.org/initiative/obesity_prevention; accessed 10/20/2014.

Bodenheimer T., Wagner EH, Grumbach K. 2002. Improving primary care for patients with chronic illness. *JAMA* 288:1775-1779.

Bochud M, Marques-Vidal P, Burnier M, Paccaud F. 2012. Dietary salt intake and cardiovascular disease: summarizing the evidence. *Pub Health Rev* 33:530-552.

Bonvecchio A., Safdie M., Monterrubio EA, Gust T., Villapando S., Rivera JA. 2009. Overweight and obesity trends in Mexican children 2 to 8 years of age from 1988–2006. *Salud Publica Mex* 51:7-12.

Boston Public Health Commission. 2011. Healthy beverage toolkit: Boston Public Health Commission. Available at: http://bphc.org/whatwedo/healthy-eating-active-living/healthy-beverages; accessed 09/10/2015.

Bourne PA. 2012. Health of children in Jamaica: the new health realities. *Indian J Med Sci* 66: 175-188.

Bourne PA. 2013. Chronic diseases, self-rated health status, health care utilization and health insurance status of males in a Caribbean nation. *J Behav Health* 2:66-78.

Bourne PA, Charles CAD. 2011. Hypertensive and modeling their social determinants of self-rated health status in a middle-income developing nation. *J Clin Diagn Res* 5:1-8.

Bourne PA, Francis C., Sharpe-Pryce C., Davis AH, Solan I. 2014a. Diabetes, hypertension, arthritis and other chronic non-communicable diseases in an English-speaking Caribbean Nation: A Health Perspective. *J Endocrinol Diab* 1:12.

Bourne PA, Francis C., Sharpe-Pryce C., Hudson-Davis A, Solan I.,Watson-Coleman, O., Rhule, J., Clarke, J., Campbell-Smith J. 2014b. Unspecified non-communicable diseases in Jamaica: Has the time come to unravel this label? *J Trop Dis* 2:138 doi:10.4172/2329-891X.1000138

Bourne PA, McDaniel S., Williams MS, Francis C., Kerr-Campbell MD, et al. 2010. The changing faces of diabetes, hypertension and arthritis in a Caribbean population. *N Am J Med Sci* 2:221-229.

Bourne PA, McDaniel S., Williams MS, Francis C., Kerr-Campbell MD, et al. 2010. The changing faces of diabetes, hypertension and arthritis in a Caribbean population. *N Am J Med Sci* 2:221-229.

Bovill EG, Silva JF, Subramanian N. 1975. An epidemiologic study of osteogenic sarcoma in Malaysia. Incidence in urban as compared with rural environments and in each of three separate racial groups, 1969-1972. *Clin Orthop Relat Res* 113:119-127.

Bradshaw D., Steyn K. 2001. Poverty and chronic diseases in South Africa. WHO:Geneva, *Technical Report.* ISBN 1-919809-17-1.

Bremer AA, Mietus-Snyder ML, Lustig RH. 2012. Toward a unifying hypothesis of metabolic syndrome. Pediatrics 129:557-570.

Briggs ADM, Kehlbacher A, Tiffin R, et al. 2013. Assessing the impact on chronic disease of incorporating the societal cost of greenhouse gases into the price of food: an econometric and comparative risk assessment modeling study. *BMJ Open* doi:10.1136/bmjopen-2013-003543

Brock, DW, Wikler, D. 2006. Ethical issues in resource allocation, research, and new product development. In: Disease Control Priorities in Developing Countries (2nd ed.). Jamison DT, Breman JG, Measham AR, et al., eds. Washington (DC): World Bank.

Brownson CA, O'Toole ML, Shetty G., Anwuri VA, Fisher EB. 2007. Clinic-community partnerships: A foundation for providing community supports for diabetes care and self-management. *Diabetes Spectrum* 20:209-214.

Butler CD, Harley D. 2010. Primary, secondary and tertiary effects of eco-climatic change: the medical response. *Postgrad Med J* 86:230-234.

Cabellero B., Popkin BM. 2002. Introduction. In: The nutrition transition: diet and disease in the developing world (B. Cabellero and BM Popkin, eds.). *Academic Press*, NY, pp. 1-5.

Caballero B. 2005. A nutrition paradox-underweight and obesity in developing countries. *N Engl J Med* 352:1514-1516.

Canadian Diabetes Association. Stats Can. Population Projections for Canada, Provinces and Territories, 2005-2031. Ottawa, ON: Stats Can. Catalogue 91-520-XWE. ISBN 0-660-60635-6. Available at: http://www.statcan.gc.ca/pub/91-520- x/00105/4095095-eng.htm. Accessed 09/07/2014.

CARICOM Secretariat. 2007. Communiqué issued at the conclusion of the regional summit of heads of government of the Caribbean Community (CARICOM) on chronic non-communicable diseases (NCDS). Port-of-Spain: Trinidad and Tobago.

Caribbean Community Secretariat [Internet]. 2013. Caribbean Cooperation in Health Phase III (CCH III): regional health framework 2010-2015. Georgetown: Caribbean Community; 2013. Available at: www.caricom.org/jsp/community; accessed 01/22/2013.

Caribbean Community Secretariat. 2011. Strategic Plan of Action for the Prevention and Conrol [sic.] of Non-communicable diseases for countries of the Caribbean Community 2011-2015. Washington & Georgetown: Pan American Health Organization & CARICOM Secretariat; 2011. Available at: www.healthycaribbean.org/publications/strategic-plan-of-action.html; accessed 01/24/2014.

Caribbean Community Secretariat. 2006a. Communiqué issued at the conclusion of the twenty-seventh meeting of the conference of heads of government of the Caribbean Community (CARICOM). Georgetown: Caribbean Community; 2006.

Caribbean Community Secretariat. 2006b. CARICOM priority necessary to lowering non-communicable diseases. Georgetown: Caribbean Community; 2006.

Carvalho AK, Menezes AMB, Camelier A., Rosa FW, Nascimento OA, Perez-Padilla R., Jardim JR. 2012. Prevalence of self-reported chronic diseases in individuals over the age of 40 in São Paulo, Brazil: the Platino study Cad. Saúde Pública 28:905-912.

Cecchini M., Sassi F., Lauer JA, Lee YY, Guajardo-Barron V., Chisholm D. 2010. Chronic diseases: Tackling of unhealthy diets, physical inactivity, and obesity: health effects and cost-effectiveness. Lancet DOI:10.1016/S0140-6736(10)61514-0. Available at: www.thelancet.com; accessed 09/05/2015

CDC (Centers for Disease Control). 2010. The CDC guide to strategies for reducing the consumption of sugar-sweetened beverages. Available at: http://www.cdph.ca.gov; accessed 09/10/2015.

CDC (Centers for Disease Control). 2015. The Social-Ecological Model: A framework for prevention. Available at: www.cdc.gov; accessed 09/28/2015

Chatterjee S., Riewpaiboon A., Piyauthakit P., Riewpaiboon W. Boupaijit K., Panpuwong, N., Archavanuntagul V. 2011. Cost of diabetes and its complications in Thailand: A complete picture of economic burden. *Health Soc Care Comm* 19:289–298.

Cheema A, Adeloye D, Sidhu S, Sridhar D, Chan KY. 2014. Urbanization and prevalence of type 2 diabetes in Southern Asia: A systematic analysis. *J Glob Health* 4. Available from: http://www.ncbi.nlm.nih.gov/pmc/articles/PMC4073245/; accessed 09/10/2015.

Chen K., Ho Y., Lai C., Tsai Y., Chen S. 2004. Trends in concentration of ground-level ozone and meteorological conditions during high ozone episodes in the Kao-Ping Airshed, Taiwan. *J. Air Waste Manag* 54:36-48.

Chen L, Hu F, Yeung E, Willett W, Zhang C. 2009. Prospective study of pre-gravid sugar-sweetened beverage consumption and the risk of gestational diabetes mellitus. *Diabetes Care* 32:2236-2241

Cisse B, Luchini S, Moatti JP. 2007. Progressivity and horizontal equity in health care finance and delivery: What about Africa? *Health Policy* 80:51–68.

Coleman K, Austin BT, Brach C, Wagner EH. 2009. Evidence on the Chronic Care Model in the new millennium. *Health Aff* (Millwood) 28:75-85.

Confalonieri U., Menne B., Akhtar R., Ebi KL, Hauengue M., Kovats RS, Revich B., Woodward A. 2007: Human health. Climate Change 2007: Impacts, adaptation and vulnerability. Contribution of Working Group II to the Fourth Assessment Report of the Intergovernmental Panel on Climate Change, M.L. Parry, O.F. Canziani, J.P. Palutikof, P.J. van der Linden and C.E. Hanson (Eds.), Cambridge University Press, Cambridge, UK, 391-431.

Cobiac LJ, Vos T, Veerman JL. Cost-effectiveness of interventions to reduce dietary salt intake. *Heart.* 2010;96:1920-5.

Commonwealth Health Online. 2015. Non-communicable diseases in Cameroon. Available at: http://www.commonwealthhealth.org; accessed 09/26/2015.

Costello A, Abbas M, Allen A, et al. 2009. Managing the health effects of climate change: Lancet and University College London Institute for Global Health Commission. *Lancet* 373:1693–733.

Cradock AL, Kenney EL, McHugh A, Conley L, Mozaffarian RS, Reiner JF, Gortmaker SL. 2015. Evaluating the impact of the healthy beverage executive order for city agencies in Boston, Massachusetts, 2011–2013. *Prev Chronic Dis* 12:140549. DOI: http://dx.doi.org/10.5888/pcd12.140549.

Cretin S, Shortell SM, Keeler EB. 2004. An evaluation of collaborative interventions to improve chronic illness care. Framework and study design. *Eval Rev* 2004; 28:28-51

Daar AS, Singer PA, Persad DL, Pramming SK, Matthews DR, Beaglehole R., Bernstein A., Borysiewicz LK. 2007. Grand challenges in chronic non-communicable diseases. *Nature* 450:494-496.

Dahly DL, Adair LS. 2007. Quantifying the urban environment: a scale measure of urbanicity outperforms the urban–rural dichotomy. *Soc Sci Med* 64:1407–1419.

Dain K., Hadley L. 2012. Diabetes and climate change: Two interconnected global challenges. *Diabetes Voice* 57:25-26.

Davy C., Bleasel J., Liu H., Tchan M., Ponniah S., Brown A. 2015. Effectiveness of chronic care models: opportunities for improving healthcare practice and health outcomes: a systematic review. *BMC Health Services Research* 15:194 DOI 10.1186/s12913-015-0854-8

De-Graft Aikins A., Unwin N., Agyemang C., Allotey P., Campbell P., Arhinful D. 2010. Tackling Africa's chronic disease burden: from the local to the global. *Globalization* Health 6:5.

de Jagar C. 2012. Chronic kidney disease on the rise. Health 24. Available at: www.health24.com/medical/kidney-and-bladder/news/chronic-kidney-disease-on-therise

de Klerk MMY. 2000. Aantal chronisch zieken en gehandicapten [Number of chronically ill and disabled] (In Dutch). In: De Klerk MMY, ed. Rapportage ouderen 2000 Arbeidsmarktpositie en financie¨ le situatie van mensen met beperkingen en/of chronische ziekten [Report on the Disabled 2000] (In Dutch). Den Haag: Sociaal en Cultureel Planbureau 25e56.

Dennill, K., King, L. and Swanepol, T. (eds.), 1998. Aspects of primary health care; community health care in Southern Africa. Oxford University Press Southern Africa: Cape Town.

Detaille SI, Heerkens YF, Engels JA, et al. 2009. Common prognostic factors of work disability among employees with a chronic somatic disease: a systematic review of cohort studies. *Scand J Work Environ Health* 35:21.

DeVol, R, Bedroussian, A, et al. 2007. *An Unhealthy America: The Economic Burden of Chronic Disease.* The Milken Institute. October 2007.

Dhingra R, Sullivan L, Jacques PF, Wang TJ, Fox CS, Meigs JB, D'Agostino RB, Gaziano JM, Vasan RS. 2007. Soft drink consumption and risk of developing cardiometabolic risk factors and the metabolic syndrome in middle-aged adults in the community. *Circulation* 116:480–488.

DiRocco A. Cuvi N. 2014. An ethnographic approach to the nutrition transition in Ecuador *J Global Health.* Available at: www.ghjournal.org/an-ethnographic-approach-to-the-nutrition-transition; accessed 10/19/2014.

Doak CM, Popkin B. 2008. The rapid emergence of obesity in developing countries. In: Nutrition and Health in Developing Countries (2nd edition). Semba RD, Bloem MW, Piot P. Totowa (eds.). NJ: Humana Press: pp. 617-638.

Donders NCGM, Bos JT, van der Velden K., van der Gulden JWJ. 2012. Age differences in the associations between sick leave and aspects of health, psychosocial workload and family life: a cross-sectional study. *BMJ Open* 2:e000960. doi:10.1136/bmjopen-2012-000960.

Drewnowski A., Darmon N. 2005. The economics of obesity: Dietary energy density and energy cost. *Am J Clin Nutr* 82:S265–73.

Drewnowski, A. and Popkin, B.M. The nutrition transition: new trends in the global diet. *Nutrition Reviews* (February 1997) 55, 2: 31-43.

Duran A., Kutzin J., Menabde N. 2014. Universal coverage challenges require health system approaches: the case of India. *Health Policy* 114:269-277.

Durstine JL, Gordon B., Wang Z., Luo X. 2013. Chronic disease and the link to physical activity. *J Sport Health* Sci 2:3-11.

Eberstadt N. 2011. The dying bear: Russia's demographic disaster. *Foreign Affairs* 90:95-108.

Globocan 2012, IARC.

Ebi KL, Exuzides KA, Lau E., et al. 2004. Weather changes associated with hospitalizations for cardiovascular diseases and stroke in California, 1983-1998. *Internat J Biometeorol* 49:48-58.

Echouffo-Tcheugui JB, Kengne, AP. 2011. Chronic non-communicable diseases in Cameroon: burden, determinants and current policies. *Globalization and Health* 7:44

Economic Intelligence Unit. 2014.

Edwards P., Roberts I. 2009. Population adiposity and climate change. *Internat J Epi* 38:1137-1140.

Egbe M. 2013. Country Report: The healthcare system of Cameroon: Socio-Economic characteristics; historical context; organizational & financial aspects; major public health programs & challenges; strength and weaknesses. *J Sustainable Reg Health System.* Available at: http://www.researchgate.net/publication/236166490; accessed 09/14/2015.

Eldemire-Shearer D, James K, Morris C, Holder-Nevins D, Lawes H, et al. 2011. Chronic disease and ageing in the Caribbean: opportunities knock at the door. *West Indian Med J* 60: 471-477.

Elrayah-Eliadarous, H. 2007. *Economic burden of diabetes on patients and their families in Sudan.* Department of Public Health Sciences, Division of International Health. Stockholm, Karolinska Institute.

Emoti CE, Enosolcase ME. 2008. The effect of accessibility to drugs on outcome of therapy in-patients with malignant lymphoma. *Niger Postgrad Med J* 15:10–14.

EO (Executive Order of Mayor Thomas M. Menino). 2011. *An order relative to healthy beverage options, city of Boston.* Available at: Boston. Available at: www.cityofboston.gov; accessed 09/10/2015.

Epping-Jordan JE, Pruitt SD, Bengoa R, Wagner EH. 2004. Improving the quality of health care for chronic conditions. *Quality and Safety in Health Care* 13:299-305.

European Commission. 2009. National Salt Initiatives Implementing the EU Framework for salt reduction initiatives.

Food Standards Agency. 2009. UK Salt Reduction Initiatives. [out of place] New York City Department of Health and Mental Hygiene. 2010. Cutting Salt, Improving Health—Packaged Food.

Ezzati M., Vander Hoorn S., Lawes C., Leach R., James W., Lopez, AD., et al. (2005). Rethinking the "Diseases of Affluence" paradigm: Global patterns of nutritional risk in relation to economic development. *PLoS Medicine* 2:e133.

Fagherazzi G., Villier A., Sartorelli S., Lajous M., Balkau B., Clavel-Chapelon F. 2013. Consumption of artificially and sugar-sweetened beverages and incident type 2 diabetes in the Etude Epidemiologique aupres des femmes de la Mutuelle Generale de l'Education Nationale-European Prospective Investigation into Cancer and Nutrition cohort. *Am J Clin Nutr* 97:517-523.

FAO (Food and Agricultural Organization). 2010. Fats and fatty acids in human nutrition: report of an expert consultation. FAO Food and Nutrition Paper 91. Food and Agricultural Organization of the United Nations, Rome.

Ferlay J, Soerjomataram I, Ervik M, Dikshit R, Eser S, Mathers C, Rebelo M, Parkin DM, Forman D, Bray, F. 2012. Cancer Incidence and Mortality Worldwide: IARC Cancer Base No. 11 [Internet]. Lyon, France: International Agency for Research on Cancer; 2013.

Ford ES, Mokdad AH. 2008. Epidemiology of obesity in the Western Hemisphere. *J Clin Endocrinol Metab* 93:S1-S8.

Fitzpatrick AL, Ngo QV, Ly KA, Ton TGN, Longstreth WT, Vo TT, Heitzinger K., Pham CH, Tirschwell DL. 2012. Symptoms and risk factors for stroke in a community-based observational sample in Viet Nam. *J Epidemiol Global Health* 2:155-163.

Ford CN, Ng S-W, Popkin BM. 2015. Targeted beverage taxes influence food and beverage purchases among households with preschool children. *J Nutr* 145:1835-1843.

Fung TT, Malik V, Rexrode KM, Manson JE, Willett WC, Hu FB. 2009. Sweetened beverage consumption and risk of coronary heart disease in women. *Am J Clin Nutr* 89:1037–1042

Gaziano TA., Pagidipati N. 2013. Scaling up chronic disease prevention interventions in lower-and middle-income countries. *Annu Rev Public Health* 34: 317–335.

GLOBOCAN 1 (Available from: http://globocan.iarc.fr, accessed on 9/13/2014).

Gómez Dantés O., Sesma S., Becerril VM, Knaul FM, Arreola H., Frenk J. 2011. Sistema de salud de México. *Salud Pública Méx* 53:220-232

Goodman RM, Wandersman A., Chinman M. et al. 1996. An ecological assessment of community-based interventions for prevention and health promotion: Approaches to measuring community coalitions. *Am J Community Psychol* 24:33-61.

Gong H., Wong R., Sarma RJ, Linn WS, Sullivan ED, Shamoo DA, Anderson KR, Prasad SB. 1998. Cardiovascular effects of ozone exposure in human volunteers. *Am J Respir Crit Care Med* 158:538-546.

Flessa S. 2003. Priorities and allocation of health care resources in developing countries: A case-study from the Mtwara region, Tanzania. *Eur J Oper Res* 150:67-80.

Godfrey R, Julien M. 2005. Urbanisation and health. *Clinical Medicine* 5:137–141.

Goudge J, Gilson L, Russell S, Gumede T, Mills A. 2009. Affordability, availability and acceptability barriers to health care for the chronically ill: longitudinal case studies from South Africa. *BMC Health Serv Res* 9:75.

Graudal NA, Hubeck-Graudal T, Jurgens G. 2011. Effects of low sodium diet versus high sodium diet on blood pressure, renin, aldosterone, catecholamines, cholesterol, and triglyceride. *Cochrane Database Syst Rev* 11:CD004022.

Gruen RL, Pearson SD, Brennan TA. 2006. Physician citizens - public roles and professional responsibilities. *JAMA* 291:94-98.

Guthold R, Ono T, Kathleen L, Strong KL, Chatterji S, Morabia A. 2008. Worldwide variability in physical inactivity: A 51-country survey. *Am J Prev Med* 34:486-94.

Guthold R., Louazani SA, Riley LM, Cowan MJ, Bovet P., Damasceno A., Sambo BH, Tesfaye F., Armstrong TP. 2011. Physical activity in 22 African countries: results from the World Health Organization STEPwise approach to chronic disease risk factor surveillance. *Am J Prev Med* 4:52-60.

Haines A., Kovats RS, Campbell-Lendrum D., Corvalan C. 2006. Climate change and human health: Impacts, vulnerability and public health. *Pub Health* 120:585-596.

Hanna TP. 2008. Radiation oncology in the developing world. In: Halperin EC, Perez CA, Brady LW (eds.). Perez and Brady's principles and practices of radiation oncology, 5th edn. Philadelphia: *Lippincott Williams & Williams*, pp. 604-610.

Hardman AE. Physical activity and cancer risk. 2006. *Proceedings of the Nutrition Society* 60:107-13.

He FJ, MacGregor GA. 2013. Effect of longer-term modest salt reduction on blood pressure. *Cochrane Database Syst Rev* 4:CD004937.

He FJ, Pombo-Rodrigues S, MacGregor GA. 2014. Salt reduction in England from 2003 to 2011: its relationship to blood pressure, stroke and ischaemic heart disease mortality. *BMJ Open* 4: (4).

Health Canada. 2010. Guidance for the food industry on reducing sodium in processing foods. Available at: www.hc-sc.gc.ca; accessed 09/07/2015.

Hennis AJ, Fraser HS, Jonnalagadda R., Fuller J., Chaturvedi N. 2004. Explanations for the high risk of diabetes-related amputation in a Caribbean population of black African descent and potential for prevention. *Diabetes Care* 27:2636-2641.

Henry CJ, Webster-Gandy J, Varakamin C. 2001. A comparison of physical activity levels in two contrasting elderly populations in Thailand. *Am J Human Biol* 1:310-15.

Henry-Lee A., Yearwood A. (1999). Protecting the poor and the medically indigent under health insurance: a case study of Jamaica. Small Appl Res #6 Bethesda, MD: Partnerships for Health Reform Project, Abt Associates Inc.

Higuchi M. 2009. Costs, availability and affordability of diabetes care in the Philippines. Foundation for Advanced Studies on International Development, 2009. Available at: www.haiweb.org/medicineprices/news/index.html. Accessed 7/13/2015

Higuchi M. 2010. Lifestyle diseases: Access to chronic disease care in low- and middle-income countries. UN Chronicle XLVII 2 2010.

Hobsbawm E. 1996. The industrial revolution. In: The Age of Revolution. *Vintage Books*, NY.

Hooper L, Abdelhamid A, Moore HJ, Douthwaite W, Skeaff CM, Summerbell CD. 2012. Effect of reducing total fat intake on body weight: systematic review and meta-analysis of randomised controlled trials and cohort studies. *BMJ* 345: e7666.

Hope KR. 1989. Managing rapid urbanization in the third world: Some aspects of policy. *Genus* 45:21-35.

Hospedales CJ, Samuels TA, Cummings R., Gollop G., Greene E. 2011. Raising the priority of chronic non-communicable diseases in the Caribbean. *Rev Panam Salud Publica* 30: 393-400.

Huang Y. 2011. The sick man of Asia: China's health crisis. *Foreign Affairs* 90:119-136.

IAS (International Atherosclerosis Society). 2015. An International Atherosclerosis Society Position Paper: Global Recommendations for the Management of Dyslipidemia. Available at: http://www.athero.org; accessed 09/05/2015.

Hummasti S., Hotamisligil GS. 2010. Endoplasmic reticulum stress and inflammation in obesity and diabetes. *Circ Res* 107:579-591.

IASO Policy Briefing. 2014. The prevention of obesity and NCDs: Challenges and opportunities for governments January 2014. Available at: http://www.worldobesity.org; accessed 9/28/2015.

Ibrahim MM, Damasceno A. 2012. Hypertension in developing countries. *Lancet* 380:611-619.

IDF (International Diabetes Federation). 2013. IDF Diabetes Atlas, 6th edition, International Diabetes Federation. Available at: www.idf.org/diabetesatlas; accessed 09/07/2014.

IDF (International Diabetes Federation). 2007. The Economic Impacts of Diabetes, Chapter 5, Diabetes Atlas, International Diabetes Federation, Brussels, Belguim.

IDF (International Diabetes Federation). 2015. IDF framework for action on sugar. Brussels, Belguim.

IFPRI (International Food Policy Research Institute). 2015. Global Nutrition Report 2015: Actions and accountability to advance nutrition and sustainable development. Available at: www.ifpri.org/publication/global-nutrition-report; accessed 09/24/2015.

INCTR (International Network for Cancer Treatment and Research). 2014. Cancer in developing countries. Available at: http://www.inctr.org/about-inctr/cancer-in-developing-countries; accessed 7/13/2015.

InterAct Consortium. 2013. Consumption of sweet beverages and type 2 diabetes incidence in European adults: results from EPIC-InterAct. *Diabetologia* 56:1520-1530.

IPCC. 2007. Climate change 2007: Impacts, adaptation, and vulnerability. In: M.L. Parry, O.F. Canziani, J.P. Palutikof, P.J. van der Linden, C.E. Hanson (eds.). Contribution of Working Group II to the fourth assessment report of the intergovernmental panel on climate change (pp. 976). Cambridge, UK: Cambridge University Press.

IRIN. 2013. Chronic lifestyle diseases strain South Africa's health system. Available at: http://www.irinnews.org; accessed 10/9/2014.

Ishine M., Wada T., Sakagami T., Dung PT, Vienh TD, Kawakita T, Fushida M, Okumiya K, Kita T, Matsubayashi K. 2005. Comprehensive geriatric assessment for community dwelling elderly in Asia compared with those in Japan: III. Phuto in Vietnam. *Geriatrics Gerontol Internat* 5:115-121.

Ishine M., Sakagami T., Sakamoto R., Wada T., Khampitak K., Fushida M., Kawakita T., Okumiya K., Kita T., Matsubayashi K. 2006. Comprehensive geriatric assessment for community dwelling elderly in Asia compared with those in Japan: VII. Khon Khen in Thailand. *Geriatrics Gerontol Internat* 6:40-48.

Islam MA, Azad AK. 2014. An increase of the health care cost of diabetes mellitus type 2: A precise review on economic impact of diabetes. *Aust J Basic Appl Sci* 8:40-44.

James J, Soyibo AK, Hurlock L., Gordon-Strachan G., Barton EN. 2012. Cardiovascular risk factors in an Eastern Caribbean Island: Prevalence of non-communicable chronic diseases and associated lifestyle risk factors for cardiovascular morbidity and mortality in the British Virgin Islands. *West Indian Med J* 61: 429-436.

Jha P., Nugent R., Verguet S., Bloom D., Hum R. 2012. Chronic disease prevention and control. Copenhagen Consensus 2012 Challenge Paper.

Jha V. Garcia-Garcia G., Iseki K., Li Z., Naicker S., Plattner B., Saran R. Wang AY-M, Yang C-W. 2013. Chronic kidney disease: global dimension and perspectives. *The Lancet* http://dx.doi.org/10.1016/S0140-6736.

John RM. 2008. Price elasticity estimates for tobacco products in India. *Health Policy Plan* 23:200–9.

Kain J., Vio F., Albala C. 2003. Obesity trends and determinant factors in Latin America. *Cad Saude Publica* 19:S77-S86.

Kautzky, K. and Tollman, S.M. 2009. A perspective on primary health care in South Africa. Health Systems Trust: South Africa.

Karppanen H., Mervaala E. 2006. Sodium intake and hypertension. *Prog Cardiovasc Dis* 49:59-75.

Kelly B, King L, Bauman A, Smith BJ, Flood V. The effects of different regulation systems on television food advertising to children. *Aust N Z J Public Health*. 2007;31:340-3

Kessler RC, Greenberg PE, Mickelson KD, Meneades LM, Wang PS. 2001. The effects of chronic medical conditions on work loss and work cutback. *J Occup Environ Med* 43:218-225.

Khowaja LA, Khuwaja AK, Cosgrove P. 2007. Cost of diabetes care in out-patient clinics of Karachi, Pakistan. *BMC Health Services Res* 7:189.

Kirigia JM, Sambo LG, Kainyu LH. 2000. Willingness to pay for schistosomiasis-related health outcomes in Kenya. *Afr J Health Sci* 7:55-67.

Kirigia JM, Sambo LG. 2003. Cost of mental and behavioural disorders in Kenya. *Ann Gen Hosp Psychiatry* 2:7.

Kirigia JM, Sambo LG, Aldis W, Mwabu G. 2004. Impact of disaster-related mortality on gross domestic product in the WHO African Region. *BMC Emerg Med* 4:1.

Kirigia JM, Sambo HB, Sambo LG, Barry SP. 2009. Economic burden of diabetes mellitus in the WHO African region. *BMC Internat Health and Hum Rights* 9:6.

Kirsh S, Watts S, Pascuzzi K, et al. 2007. Shared medical appointments based on the chronic care model: a quality improvement project to address the challenges of patients with diabetes with high cardiovascular risk. *Qual Saf Health Care* 16:349 –53.

Kolbe-Alexander TL, Lambert EV, Charlton KE. 2006. Effectiveness of a community based low intensity exercise program for older adults. *J Nutr Health Aging* 10:21- 9.

Koning L de, Malik VS, Rimm EB, Willett WC, Hu FB. 2011. Sugar-sweetened and artificially sweetened beverage consumption and risk of type 2 diabetes in men. *Am J Clin Nutr*. 93:1321–7.

Knaul FM and Frenk J. 2005. Health insurance in Mexico: achieving universal coverage through structural reform. *Health Aff* (Millwood) 24:1467-1476.

Knaul FM, González-Pier E, Gómez-Dantés O, García-Junco D, Arreola-Ornelas H, Barraza-Llorens M, Sandoval R, Caballero F, Hernández M, Juan M, Kershenobich D, Nigenda G, Ruelas E, Sepulveda J, Tapia R, Soberón G, Chertorivski S, Frenk J. 2012. The quest for universal health coverage: Achieving social protection for all in Mexico. *Lancet* 380:1259-1279.

Krewski D., Jerrett M., Burnett RT, Ma R., Hughes E., Shi Y., Turner MC, Pope CA, Thurston G. et al. 2009. Extended follow-up and spatial analysis of the American Cancer Society study linking particulate air pollution and mortality. *Res Rep Health Eff* 140:5-114.

Kruger HS, Venter CS, Vorster HH, Margetts BM. 2002. Physical inactivity is the major determinant of obesity in black women in the North West Province, South Africa: the THUSA study. *Nutrition* 8:422-27.

Kulic J. 2013. Reducing the economic burden of non-communicable diseases in BRICS: Lessons from Brazil. http://www.brics.utoronto.ca (accessed 1/14/14).

Kuwait News Agency. 2014. Health Ministry praises Kuwait firm's reduction of salt in bread and salt. 2014. Available at: (http://www.kuna.net.kw; accessed 09/08/2015.

Kysely J., Pokorna N. Kync J., Kriz B. 2009. Excess cardiovascular mortality associated with cold spells in the Czech Republic. *BMC Public Health* 9:19.

Leber R. 2014. Climate change is already causing asthma. Cancer too. New Republic. Available at: www.newrepublic.com/.../national-climate-assessment; accessed 9/14/14.

Lee I-M, Shiroma EJ, Lobelo F., Puska, P., Blair SN, Katzmarzyk PT. 2012. Effect of physical inactivity on major non-communicable diseases worldwide: an analysis of burden of disease and life expectancy. *Lancet* 380:219-229.

Lee V, Mikkelsen L, Srikantharajah J et al. 2008. Promising strategies for creating healthy eating and active living environments.

Leor J., Poole WK, Kloner RA. 1996. Sudden cardiac death triggered by an earthquake. *N Engl J Med* 334:413-419.

Levitt N. S., Steyn K., De Wet T., Morrell C., Edwards P. R., Ellison G. T. H., Cameron N. 1999. An Inverse Relation between Blood Pressure and Birth Weight among 5-Year-Old Children from Soweto, South Africa (Birth-to-Ten Study) *Journal of Epidemiology and Community Health* 53:264–68.

Lewis T., Synowiec C., Lagomarsino G., Schweitzer J. 2012. E-health in low- and middle-income countries: findings from the Center for Health Market Innovations. *Bull World Health Org* 90:332-340.

Lim SS, Vos T, Flaxman AD, Danaei G, Shibuya K, Adair-Rohani H et al. 2012. A comparative risk assessment of burden of disease and injury attributable to 67 risk factors and risk factor clusters in 21 regions, 1990-2010: a systematic analysis for the global burden of disease study 2010. *Lancet* 380:2224-2260.

Lim TO, Looi HW, Harun K., Marzida. 1991. Descriptive analysis of total medical admissions and common medical disorders in 1987 Kuantan General Hospital, using computerized inpatients' discharge record. *Med J Malays* 46:239-246.

Limb M. 2013. Public health body quits responsibility deal over government's failure to act on tobacco and alcohol. BMJ 347:f4590.

Maantay J., Becker S. 2012. The health impacts of global climate change: A geographic perspective. *Appl Geography* 33:1-3.

Magawa R. 2012. Primary healthcare implementation: A brief review. Available at: www.consultancyafrica.com; accessed 09/14/2015.

Magnussen, L., Ehiri, J. and Jolly, P. 2004. Comprehensive versus selective primary health care: Lessons for global health policy. *Health Affairs* 23:167-176.

Malik VS, Popkin BM, Bray GA, Després J-P, Hu FB. 2010. Sugar-sweetened beverages, obesity, type 2 diabetes mellitus, and cardiovascular disease risk. *Circulation* 121:1356–64.

Mathers CD, Loncar D. 2006. Projections of global mortality and burden of disease from 2002 to 2030. *PLoS Med* 3:e442.

Mathers CD, Boerma T., Ma Fat D. 2009. Global and regional causes of death. *Br Med Bull* 92:7-32.

Matsudo SM, Matsudo VR, Araujo TM, Andrade DR, Andrade EL, de Oliveira LC, Braggion GF. 2003. The Agita São Paulo program as a model for using physical activity to promote health. *Pan Am J Public Health* 14:265-72.

Mayer-Foulkes D. 2011. A survey of macro damages from non-communicable chronic diseases: Another challenge for global governance. Global Econ J 11:1.

Mayosi BM, Flisher AJ, Lalloo UG, Sitas F., Tollman SM, et al. 2009. The burden of noncommunicable diseases in South Africa. *Lancet* 374: 934-447.

Mbanya JC, Kengne AP, Assah F. 2006. Diabetes care in Africa. *Lancet* 368:1628–1629.

McGeehin MA, Mirabelli M. 2001. The potential impacts of climate variability and change on temperature-related morbidity and mortality in the United States. *Environ Health Perspect* 109 (Suppl. 2):185–189.

Mendis S, Fukino K, Cameron A, et al. 2007. The availability and affordability of selected essential medicines for chronic diseases in six low- and middle-income countries. *Bull World Health Organ* 85:279–88.

Ministerio de Salud Argentina. 2012. Argentine initiative to reduce salt consumption. Available at: http://www.paho.org/panamericanforum; accessed 09/08/20155 November 2014.

MOH (Ministry of Health). 2015. How the Green Prescription works. Available at: http://www.health.govt.nz/our-work/preventative-health-wellness/physical-activity/green-prescriptions/how-green-prescription-works; accessed 09/23/2015.

Mohan V., Seedat YK, Pradeepa R. 2013. The rising burden of diabetes and hypertension in Southeast Asian and African Regions: Need for effective strategies for prevention and control in primary health care settings. *Internat J Hypertension.* Avaialable at: http://dx.doi.org/10.1155/2013/409083

Mokhtar N, Elati J, Chabir R, Bour A, Elkari K, Schlossman NP, Caballero-B, Aguenaou-H. 2001. Diet culture and obesity in northern Africa. *J Nutr* 13:887S-92S.

Moore M, Gould P, Keary BS. 2003. Global urbanization and impact on health. *Internat J Hygiene Environ Health* 206:269–278.

Morhason-Bello IO, Odedina F., Rebbeck TR, Harford J., Dangou J-M, Denny L., Adewole IF. 2013. Challenges and opportunities in cancer control in Africa: a perspective from the African Organisation for Research and Training in Cancer. *Lancet Oncol* 14:e142-e151.

Mozaffarian D., Fahimi S., Singh GM, Micha R., Khatibzadeh S., Engell RE, Lim S., Danaei G., Ezzati M., Powles J. 2014. Global sodium consumption and death from cardiovascular causes *N Engl J Med* 371:624-634.

Muir PS. 1999. Stratospheric ozone depletion. Available at: http://people.oregonstate.edu; accessed 9/15/2014.

Murray CJL, Lopez AD. 1996. The global burden of disease. Boston, Mass: Harvard School of Public Health.

Myo Thet H., Thein N., Nyan T., May Mon K. 1992. Prevalence of cardiovascular diseases in rural area of Hmawbi and urban Yangon city. *Asia Pac J Public Health* 6:188-194.

Nagai Y. Yonemitsu S., Erion DM, Iwasaki T. Stark R. et al. 2009. The role of peroxisome proliferator-activated receptor gamma coactivator-I beta in the pathogenesis of fructose-induced insulin resistance. *Cell Metab* 9:252-264.

NCD Alliance. 2010. Non-communicable disease: The hidden epidemic….(find website)

NHI. 2011. National Health Insurance in South Africa: Policy paper', Department of Health, Republic of South Africa. Available at: http://images.businessday.co.za; accessed 09/14/2015.

Nettleton JA, Lutsey PL, Wang Y, Lima JA, Michos ED, Jacobs DR Jr. 2009. Diet soda intake and risk of incident metabolic syndrome and type 2 diabetes in the Multi-Ethnic Study of Atherosclerosis (MESA). Diabetes Care 32:688–694.

Ng SW, Norton EC, Popkin BM. 2009. Why have physical activity levels declined among Chinese adults? Findings from the 1991–2006 China Health and Nutrition Surveys. *Soc Sci Med* 68:1305–1314.

Nguyen S, Choi HK, Lustig RH, Hsu CY. 2009. Sugar-sweetened beverages, serum uric acid, and blood pressure in adolescents. *J Pediatr* 154:807–813.

Nikolic IA, Stanciole AE, Mikhail Zaydman M. 2011. Chronic Emergency: Why NCDs matter? *World Bank Health, Nutrition and Population Discussion Paper.*

Nugent R. 2008. Chronic diseases in developing countries: Health and economic burdens. *Ann NY Acad Sci* 1136:70-79.

Nishida C, Uauy R. 2009. WHO scientific update on health consequences of trans fatty acids: introduction. *Eur J Clin Nutr* 63 (Suppl 2):S1–4.

Nutting PA, Dickinson WP, Dickinson LM, Nelson CC, King DK, Crabtree BF, Glasgow RE. 2007. Use of chronic care model elements is associated with higher-quality care for diabetes. *Ann Fam Med* 5: 14-20.

Oakley P: Community involvement in health development: An examination of critical issues. Geneva: *World Health Organization* 1989.

Oboimbo, E. M., 2003. Primary health care, selective or comprehensive, which way to go? *East AfricaMedical Journal* 80:7-9.

Ockene JK, Schneider KL, Lemon SC, Ockene IS. 2011. Can we improve adherence to preventive therapies for cardiovascular health. *Circulation* 124:1276-1282.

Pan American Health Organization/Caribbean Community. 2006. Report of the Caribbean Commission on Health and Development.

PAHO (Pan American Health Organization). 2009. Health situation in the Americas: basic indicators. Washington, DC: PAHO; 2009. Available at: http://new.paho.org; accessed 09/26/2015.

PAHO (Pan American Health Organization). 2013a. Innovative care for chronic conditions: organizing and delivering high quality care for chronic noncommunicable diseases in the Americas. Washington, DC: PAHO, 2013.

PAHO (Pan American Health Organization). 2013b. Salt-smart Americas: a guide for country-level action. 2013. Washington (DC): Pan American Health Organization. Available at: http://www.paho.org; accessed 09/08/2015.

Panjwani C, Caraher M. 2013. The public health responsibility deal: Brokering a deal for public health, but on whose terms? *Health Policy* Nov 17. [Epub ahead of print].

Parchman ML, Pugh JA, Wang CP, Romero RL. 2007a. Glucose control, self-care behaviors, and the presence of the chronic care model in primary care clinics. *Diabetes Care* 30:2849 –54.

Parchman ML, Zeber JE, Romero RR, Pugh JA. 2007b. Risk of coronary artery disease in type 2 diabetes and the delivery of care consistent with the chronic care model in primary care settings: a STARNet study. *Med Care* 45:1129 –34.

Pattaya Mail. 2012. Campaign to reduce Thais' salt consumption by half. Available at http://www. pattayamail.com/news; accessed 09/08/2015.

Patz JA, Campbell-Lendrum D., Holloway T., Foley JA. 2006. Impact of regional climate change on human health. *Nature* 438:310-317.

Petticrew M et al. 2013. The public health responsibility deal: how should such a complex public health policy be evaluated? *J Public Health* (Oxf) 35:495-501.

Plumb J., Carson WLC, Rickie B., Kevin S. 2012. Community-based partnerships for improving chronic disease management. Department of Family & Community Medicine Faculty Papers. Paper 29. Available at: http://jdc.jefferson.edu/fmfp/29; accessed 09/29/2015.

Popkin BM, Horton SH, Soowon K. 2001. The nutrition transition and prevention of diet-related diseases in Asia and the Pacific. *Food Nutr Bull* 22:S4. United Nations University Press.

Popkin BM. 2002. The shift in stages of the nutrition transition in the developing world differs from past experiences! *Pub Health Nutr* 5:205-214.

Popkin B. 2003. The Nutrition Transition in the Developing World. *Development Policy Review,* 21, 581-597.

Popkin BM, Gordon-Larsen P. 2004. The nutrition transition: worldwide obesity dynamics and their determinants. *Intl J Obes* 28:S2–S9.

Portier CJ, Thigpen TK, Carter SR, Dilworth CH Grambsch AE, Gohike J., Hess J., Howard SN, Luber G., Lutz JT, Masalak T., Prudent N. et al. 2010. A human health perspective on climate change: A report outlining the research needs on human health effects of climate change. Research Triangle Park, N.C. Environmental Health Perspectives/ National Institute of Environmental Health Sciences.

Powles J., Fahimi S., Micha R., Shatibzadeh S., Shi P., Ezzati M., Engell RE, Lim SS, Danaei G., Mozaffarian D. 2013. Global, regional and national sodium intakes in 1990 and 2010: a systematic analysis of 24 h urinary sodium excretion and dietary surveys worldwide. *BMJ* Open:doi:10.1136/bmjopen-2013-003733.

Reddy SP, Panday S, Swart D, Jinabhai CC, Amosun SL, James S, et al. 2003. Umthenthc uhlaba usamila - The South African youth risk behavior survey 2002. Cape Town: South African Medical Research Council. Available at www.mrc.ac.za/healthpromotion; accessed 09/05/2015.

Reinivuo H., Valsta LM, Laatikainen T., Tuomilehto J., Pietinen P. 2006. Sodium in the Finnish diet: II Trends in dietary sodium intake and comparison between intake and 24-h excretion of sodium. *Eur J Clin Nutr* 60:1160-7.

Riewpaiboon A., Pornlertwadee P., Pongsawat K. 2007. Diabetes cost model of a hospital in Thailand. *Value Health* 10:223-230.

Ritenbaugh C, Teufel-Shone NI, Aickin MG, et al. 2003. A lifestyle intervention improves plasma insulin levels among Native American high school youth. *Prev Med* 36:309-319.

Rojas-Martínez R., Aguilar-Salinas CA, Jimenez-Corona A., Gómez-Pérez FJ, Barquera S., Lazcano-Ponce E. 2012. Prevalence of obesity and metabolic syndrome components in Mexican adults without type II diabetes or hypertension. *Salud Publica Mex* 54:7-12.

Sadler K., Nicholson S., Steer T., Gill V., Bates B., Tipping S., et al. 2011. National Diet & Nutrition Survey: Assessment of dietary sodium in adults (aged 19 to 64 years) in England, 2011. Department of Health. Available: https://www.gov.uk/government/uploads/system/uploads/attachment_data/file/213420/Sodium-Survey-England-2011_Text_to-DH_FINAL1.pdf.

Samb B., Desai N., Nishtar S., Mendis S., Bekedam H., Wright A., Hsu J., Martiniuk A., Celletti F., Patel K., Adshead F., McKee M., Evans T., Alwan A., Etienne C. 2010. Prevention and management of chronic disease: a litmus test for health systems strengthening in low-income and middle-income countries. *Lancet* 376:1785-1797.

Samuels TA, Kirton J., Guebert J. 2014. Monitoring compliance with high-level commitments in health: the case of the CARICOM Summit on Chronic Non-Communicable Diseases. *Bulletin of the World Health Organization* 92:270-276B.

Santos CX, Tanaka LY, Wosniak J. Laurindo FR. 2009. Mechanisms and implications of reactive oxygen species generation during the unfolded protein response: role of endoplasmic reticulum oxidoreductases, mitochondrial electron transport, and NADPH oxidase. *Antioxid Redox Signal* 11:2409-2427.

Sassi F, Cecchini M, Lauer J, Chisholm D. Improving lifestyles, tackling obesity: the health and economic impact of prevention strategies. OECD Health working paper 48. Paris: OECD, 2009. Available at: www.who.int/choice/publications/d_OECD; accessed 09/05/2015.

Schmidt MI et al. 2011. Chronic non-communicable diseases in Brazil: Burden and current challenges. *Lancet* 6736:1-6.

Schmittdiel J, Mosen DM, Glasgow RE, Hibbard J, Remmers C, Bellows J. Patient. 2008. Assessment of Chronic Illness Care (PACIC) and improved patient-centered outcomes for chronic conditions. *J Gen Intern* Med 23:77– 80.

Schuftan C. 1999. Equity in health and economic globalisation. *Dev Pract* 9:610-614.

Schulze MB, Manson JE, Ludwig DS, Colditz GA, Stampfer MJ, Willett WC, Hu FB. 2004. Sugar-sweetened beverages, weight gain, and incidence of type 2 diabetes in young and middle-aged women. *JAMA* 292:927–934.

Schwartz J., Samet JM, Patz JA. 2004. Hospital admissions for heart disease: the effects of temperature and humidity. *Epidemiol* 15:755–761.

Shobhana R., Rama RP, Lavanya A., Williams R., Vijay V., Ramachandran A. 2000. Expenditure on health care incurred by diabetic subjects in a developing country – a study from Southern India. *Diabetes Res Clin Prac* 48:37-42.

Shokrvash B., Jamlessi F., Montazeri A., Nedjat S., Rahim A., Djazayeri A., Shojaeezadeh D. 2013. Correlates of physical activity in adolescence: a study from a developing country. Global Health Action [S.l.]:6 ISSN 1654-9880. Available at: <http://www.globalhealth action.net>; accessed: 09/23/2015.

Simarak S., de Jong UW, Breslow N., Dahl CJ, Ruckphaopunt K., Scheelings P., Maclennan R. 1977. Cancer of the oral cavity, pharynx/larynx and lung in North Thailand: case-control study and analysis of cigar smoke. *Br J Cancer* 36:130-140.

Singh GM; Micha R., Katibzadeh S., Lim S., Majid Ezzati M., Mozaffarian D. 2015. Estimated Global, Regional, and National Disease Burdens Related to Sugar-Sweetened Beverage Consumption in 2010 *Circulation* 132:639-666.

Smith KR, Woodward A., Campbell-Lendrum D., Chadee D., Honda Y., Qiyong LQ, Olwoch J., Revich B., Sauerborn R. 2014. Human health: Impacts, adaptation, and co-benefits. In: Climate change 2014: Impacts, adaptation, and vulnerability. Contribution of Working Group II to the Fifth Assessment Report of the Intergovernmental Panel on Climate Change. Intergovernmental Panel on Climate Change Cambridge University Press, Cambridge, United Kingdom and New York, NY, USA, pp. 709-754.

Sobngwi E, Mbanya JC, Unwin NC, Kengne AP, Fezeu L, Minkoulou EM, Aspray TJ, Alberti KG. 2002. Physical activity and its relationship with obesity, hypertension and diabetes in urban and rural Cameroon. *Int J Obes Relat Metab Disord* 26:1009–1016.

Solomons NW, Gross R. 1995. Urban nutrition in developing countries. *Nutr Rev* 369:39-48.

Smith KR, Jerrett M., Anderson HR, Burnett RT, Stone V., Derwent R. et al. 2009. Public health benefits of strategies to reduce greenhouse-gas emissions: Health implications of short-lived greenhouse pollutants. *Lancet* 374:2091-2103.

Sobngwi E., Mbanya JCN, Unwin NC, Terrence JA, Alberti KGM. 2001. Development and validation of a questionnaire for the assessment of physical activity in epidemiological studies in Sub-Saharan Africa. *Internat J Epidemiol* 30:1361–68.

Starfield, B. 2001. New paradigms for quality in primary care. *Br J General Prac* 51:303–9.

Stephan C, Satterthwaite D. 2008. Urban health in developing countries. *Internat Encyclopedia Pub Health* 452–463.

Stewart BW, Wild CP (eds.). 2015. World Cancer Report 2014. Available at: http://www.iarc.fr/en/publications/books/wcr/; accessed 09/01/2015.

Steyn K., Bradshaw D., Norman R., Laubscher R. 2003. Determinants and treatment of hypertension in South Africa during 1998. The first demographic and health survey (draft). Tygerburg, South Africa. South Africa Medical Research Council.

Steyn NP. 2006. Nutrition and chronic diseases of lifestyle in South Africa. In: Steyn K, Fourie J, Temple N, edn. Chronic diseases of lifestyle in South Africa: 1995-2005, Technical report, Cape Town: South African Medical Research Council. Available at: www.mrc.ac.za; accessed 09/05/2015.

Steyn NP, Senekal M, Brits S, Nel J. 2001. Urban and rural differences in dietary intake, weight status and nutrition knowledge of black female students. *Asia Pac J Clin Nutr* 9:53-9.

Stokols, D. 1996. Translating social ecological theory into guidelines for community health promotion. *Am J Health Promotion* 10:282-293.

Stuckler D. 2008. Population causes and consequences of leading chronic diseases: A comparative analysis of prevailing explanations. *The Milbank Quarterly* 86:273–326.

Stuckler D, Basu S, McKee M. 2010. Drivers of inequality in Millennium Development Goal progress: a statistical analysis. *PLoS Med* 2010; 7: e1000241 [PMID: 20209000 DOI: 10.1371/journal. pmed.1000241].

Stuckler D., Siegel K. 2012. Sick Societies: Responding to the global challenge of chronic disease. Published to Oxford Scholarship Online: January 2012 DOI: 10.1093/acprof:oso/9780199574407.001.0001

Sturchio JL. 2014. Five smart ways for the private sector and NGOS to tackle chronic diseases together. Available at: https://www.clintonfoundation.org; accessed 09/28/2015.

Su TT, Kouyate B., Flessa S. (2006). Catastrophic household expenditure for health care in a low-income society: a study from Nouna District, Burkina Faso. *Bull World Health Organ* 84:21-27.

Suhrcke M., Nugent RA, Stuckler D., Rocco L. 2006. Chronic disease: An economic perspective. London: Oxford Health Alliance. Available at: www.oxha.org; accessed 9/5/14.

Suzuki S., Sakamoto S., Koide M., Fujita H., Sakuramoto H., Kuroda T., Kintaka T., Matsuo T. 1997. Hanshin-Awaji earthquake as a trigger for acute myocardial infarction. *Am Heart J* 134:974-977.

Taimela S, Laara¨ E, Malmivaara A, et al. 2007. Self-reported health problems and sickness absence in different age groups predominantly engaged in physical work. *Occup Environ Med* 64:739e46.

Tchoumi JCT, Butera G. 2013. Profile of cardiac diagnosis in Cameroon and impact on healthcare services. *Cardiovascular Diag Ther* 3: doi: 10.3978/j.issn.2223-3652.2013. 12.05.

Teff KL, Grudziak J., Townsend RR, Dunn TN, Grant RW, et al. 2009. Endocrine and metabolic effects of consuming fructose- and glucose-sweetened beverages with meals in obese men and women: influence of insulin resistance on plasma triglyceride responses. *J Endocrinol Metab* 94:1562-1569.

The Economist Intelligence Unit. 2014. Sub-Saharan African healthcare: the user experience. A focus on non-communicable diseases.

Triggle N. 2011. Health groups reject 'responsibility deal' on alcohol. BBC News Online 14/3/2011. Available at://www.bbc.co.uk/news/health; accessed 01/10/2014.

Uauy R, Albala C, Kain J. 2001. Obesity trends in Latin America: transitioning from under to overweight. *J Nutr* 131:893S-900S.

Trieu K., Bruce Neal B., Hawkes C., Dunford E., Campbell N., Rodriguez-Fernandez R., Legetic B., McLaren L., Barberio A., Webster J. 2015. Salt Reduction Initiatives around the World – A systematic review of progress towards the global target. *PLoS ONE* 10(7): e0130247. doi:10.1371/journal.pone.0130247.

UK Department for International Development Human Development Resource Centre. 2011. Helpdesk Report: Salt intake.

UN (United Nations). 2008. World Urbanization Prospects: The 2007 Revision Population. ESA/P/WP/205 In. New York: Population Division, Department of Economic and Social Affairs, United Nations.

United Nations Population Division. 2013. Department of Economic and Social Affairs of the United Nations Secretariat (2013). *World Population Prospects: The 2012 Revision.* New York: United Nations.

U.S. Chamber of Commerce and Partnership for Prevention. 2007. *Leading by example: Leading practices for employee health management.* 2007. Accessed at: http://www.prevent.org.

Van Rompay MI, McKeown NM, Goodman E., Eliasziw M., Chomitz VR, Gordon CM, Economos CD, Sacheck JM. 2015. Sugar-sweetened beverage intake is positively associated with baseline triglyceride concentrations, and changes in intake are inversely associated with HDL cholesterol increases over 12 months in a multi-ethnic sample of children. *J Nutr* doi: 10.3945/jn.115.212662.

Venkitachalam L, Wang K., Porath A., Corbalan R., Hirsch AT, Cohen DJ, Smith SC, Ohman EM, Steg G., Bhatt EA, Magnuson EA. 2012. Global variation in the prevalence of elevated cholesterol in outpatients with established vascular disease or 3 cardiovascular risk factors according to national indices of economic development and health system performance. *Circulation* 125:1858-1864.

Villareal-Rios EA, Medina-Jauregui A., Garza-Elizondo ME, Nunez-Rocha G., Chuy-Diaz ER. 2000. The cost of diabetes mellitus and its impact on healthcare spending in Mexico. *Archives Med Res* 31:511-514.

Vlahov D, Galea S. 2002. Urbanization, urbanicity, and health. *J Urban Health* 79 (Suppl 1):S1–S12.

Wada T., Okumiy K., Suzuki K., Roriz-Cruz M., Ishine M., Sakagami T., Kita T., Matsubayashi K. 2005a. Comprehensive geriatric assessment for community-dwelling elderly in Asia compared with those in Japan: VI. Maubin in Myanmar. *Geriatrics Gerontol Internat* 5:276-285.

Wada T., Wada C., Ishine M., Okumiya K., Kawakita T., Fushida M., Kita T., Mizuno K., Matsubayashi K. 2005b. Comprehensive geriatric assessment for community dwelling elderly in Asia compared with those in Japan: V. West Java in Indonesia. *Geriatrics Gerontol Internat* 5:168-175.

Wagner EH, Austin BT, Davis C, Hindmarsh M, Schaefer J, Bonomi A. 2001. Improving chronic illness care: translating evidence into action. *Health Aff* (Millwood) 20:64–78.

Wagner EH, Davis C, Schaefer J, Von Korff M, Austin B. 1999. A survey of leading chronic disease management programs: are they consistent with the literature? *Manag Care Q*;7:56–66.

Wang M, Yu M, Fang L Ying R. 2015. Association between sugar-sweetened beverages and type 2 diabetes: A meta-analysis *J Diabetes Invest* 6:360–366.

Watanabe M., Kodama Y., Okura Y., Aizawa N., Tanabe M., Chinushi Y., Nakamura T., Nagai M., Okabe SM. 2005. Impact of earthquakes on Takotsubo cardiomyopathy. *JAMA* 294:305–307.

Webb GJ, Egger G. 2013. Obesity and climate change: can we link the two and can we deal with both together? *Am J Lifestyle Med* September 12.

Weeratunga P, Jayasinghe S, Perera Y, Jayasena G, Jayasinghe S. 2014. Per capita sugar consumption and prevalence of diabetes mellitus – global and regional associations. *BMC Public Health* 14:186.

Wilcox S., Dowda M., Griffin SF, Rheaume C., Ory MG, Leviton L., King AC, Dunn A., Buchner DM, Bazzarre T., Estabrooks PA, Campbell-voytal K., Bartlett-Prescott J., Dowdy D., Castro CM, Carpenter RA, Dzewaltowski DA, Mockenhaupt R. 2006. Results of the first year of active for life: translation of 2 evidence-based physical activity programs for older adults into community settings. *Am J Public Health* 96:1201–1209.

Wilks R., Younger N., Tulloch-Reid M., McFarlane S., Francis D. 2008. Jamaica health and lifestyle survey 2007-8. Technical Report. Kingston: Epidemiology Research Unit, Tropical Medicine Research Institute, University of the West Indies, Mona.

Winkelmayer WC, Stampfer MJ, Willett WC, Curhan GC. 2005. Habitual caffeine intake and the risk of hypertension in women. *JAMA* 294:2330–2335.

World Economic Forum, Harvard School of Public Health. 2011. From burden to "best buys": Reducing the economic impact of NCDs in low- and middle – income countries. Available at: www.weforum.org/EconomicsofNCD; accessed 12/01/2014.

WHO (World Health Organization). 2000. Health systems: Improving performance. The World Health Report 2000. World Health Organization, Geneva.
WHO (World Health Organization). 2002a. The World Health Report 2002. Geneva, World Health Organization.
WHO (World Health Organization). 2002b. Innovative care for chronic conditions: building blocks for action. Geneva: WHO; 2002. Available at:ww.who.int/chp; accessed July 29, 2015.
WHO (World Health Organization). 2004. The global burden of disease: 2004 update. Geneva, World Health Organization.
WHO (World Health Organization). 2005a. WHO: Preventing chronic disease. A vital investment. Geneva, WHO.
WHO (World Health Organization). 2005b. Health effects of transport-related air pollution (eds. Krzyzanowski et al.). Copenhagen, World Health Organisation Regional Office for Europe.
WHO (World Health Organization). 2006. WHO air quality guidelines for particulate matter, ozone, nitrogen dioxide and sulphur dioxide: Global update 2005. Geneva, WHO.
WHO (World Health Organization). 2008. The World Health Report 2008 - primary health care (Now More Than Ever). The World Health Report 2008. World Health Organization, Geneva.
WHO (World Health Organization). 2009. Climate change exposures, chronic diseases and mental health in urban populations: A threat to health security, particularly for the poor and disadvantaged. WHO Centre for Health Development.
WHO (World Health Organization). 2010. Global forum to improve developing country access to medical devices. Available at: www.who.int/mediacentre; accessed 07/13/15.
WHO (World Health Organization). 2011a. Global status report on non-communicable diseases 2010. Geneva, World Health Organization.
WHO (World Health Organization). 2011b. Global atlas on cardiovascular disease prevention and control. Geneva, World Health Organization.
WHO (World Health Organization). 2012a. World health statistics, 2012, Geneva, World Health Organization.
WHO (World Health Organization). 2012b. Guideline: Potassium intake for adults and children. Geneva, World Health Organization.
WHO (World Health Organization). 2013. Global action plan for the prevention and control of non-communicable diseases 2013-2020. Geneva, World Health Organization. Available at www.who.int; accessed 12/01/2014.
Global status report on non-communicable diseases 2014a. Geneva, World Health Organization.
(WHO) World Health Organization. 2014b. Non-communicable diseases (ncd) country profiles. Available at: http://www.who.int/nmh/countries; accessed 09/15/2015.
WHO (World Health Organization). 2015. Guideline: Sugars intake for adults and children. Geneva, World Health Organization.
WHO and Healthcare without Harm. 2009. Healthy hospitals, healthy planet, healthy people: Addressing climate change in healthcare settings. Available at http://www.who.int/globalchange/publications/healthcare_settings/en/
WHO (World Health Organization). WHO Global InfoBase. Available at: https://apps.who.int/infobase/Index.aspx (accessed March 12, 2012).

Williams GC, Lynch M, Glasgow RE. 2010. Computer assisted intervention improves patient-centered diabetes care by increasing autonomy support. Health Psychol 2007;26:728 –34.

Woolf S. 2000. Social policy and health policy. *JAMA* 11:1166-1169.

World Bank. 2015. Health expenditure, total (% of GDP). Available at: http://data.worldbank.org/indicator/SH.XPD.TOTL.ZS; accessed 09/01/2015.

Woteki CE, Thomas PR (Eds). 1992. Eat for Life: The Food and Nutrition Board's guide to reducing your risk of chronic disease. Institute of Medicine (US) Committee on Diet and Health. Washington (DC): National Academies Press (US).

Wu-Chang SJH, Chiang S-S, Chen H-F, Shih-Tzer Tsai S-H. 2001. The impact of diabetes on economics costs in dialysis patients: Experience in Taiwan. *Diabetes Res Clin Prac* 54:S47-S54.

Yamauchi T., Umezaki M., Ohtsuka R. 2001. Influence of urbanisation on physical activity and dietary changes in Huli-speaking population: A comparative study of village dwellers and migrants in urban settlements. *Br J Nutr* 85:65-73.

Young F., Critchley JA, Johnstone LK, Unwin NC. 2009. A review of co-morbidity between infectious and chronic diseases in Sub Saharan Africa: TB and diabetes mellitus, HIV, and metabolic syndrome, and the impact of globalization. *Globalization & Health* 5:9.

Zawiah, D. 2007. Direct costs of treating diabetic foot in orthopaedic ward, Hospital University Sains Malaysia. Department of Community Medicine. Kelantan, Universiti Sains Malaysia Library (Master Dissertation).

Zerbe L. 2014. It's official: Air pollution causes cancer. Available at: www. rodalenews.com/air-pollution-causes-cancer; accessed 10/12/2014.

Appendix A

Sustainable Development Goals

(http://www.un.org/sustainabledevelopment/sustainable-development-goals)

Goal 1: End Poverty in All Its Forms Everywhere

Targets

- By 2030, eradicate extreme poverty for all people everywhere, currently measured as people living on less than $1.25 a day 1.2
- By 2030, reduce at least by half the proportion of men, women and children of all ages living in poverty in all its dimensions according to national definitions
- Implement nationally appropriate social protection systems and measures for all, including floors, and by 2030 achieve substantial coverage of the poor and the vulnerable
- By 2030, ensure that all men and women, in particular the poor and the vulnerable, have equal rights to economic resources, as well as access to basic services, ownership and control over land and other forms of 13 property, inheritance, natural resources, appropriate new technology and financial services, including microfinance
- By 2030, build the resilience of the poor and those in vulnerable situations and reduce their exposure and vulnerability to climate-related extreme events and other economic, social and environmental shocks and disasters
- Ensure significant mobilization of resources from a variety of sources, including through enhanced development cooperation, in order to provide adequate and predictable means for developing countries, in particular least developed countries, to implement programs and policies to end poverty in all its dimensions
- Create sound policy frameworks at the national, regional and international levels, based on pro-poor and gender-sensitive development strategies, to support accelerated investment in poverty eradication actions.

Goal 2: End Hunger, Achieve Food Security and Improved Nutrition and Promote Sustainable Agriculture

- By 2030, end hunger and ensure access by all people, in particular the poor and people in vulnerable situations, including infants, to safe, nutritious and sufficient food all year round
- By 2030, end all forms of malnutrition, including achieving, by 2025, the internationally agreed targets on stunting and wasting in children under 5 years of age, and address the nutritional needs of adolescent girls, pregnant and lactating women and older persons
- By 2030, double the agricultural productivity and incomes of small-scale food producers, in particular women, indigenous peoples, family farmers, pastoralists and fishers, including through secure and equal access to land, other productive resources and inputs, knowledge, financial services, markets and opportunities for value addition and non-farm employment
- By 2030, ensure sustainable food production systems and implement resilient agricultural practices that increase productivity and production, that help maintain ecosystems, that strengthen capacity for adaptation to climate change, extreme weather, drought, flooding and other disasters and that progressively improve land and soil quality
- By 2020, maintain the genetic diversity of seeds, cultivated plants and farmed and domesticated animals and their related wild species, including through soundly managed and diversified seed and plant banks at the national, regional and international levels, and promote access to and fair and equitable sharing of benefits arising from the utilization of genetic resources and associated traditional knowledge, as internationally agreed
- Increase investment, including through enhanced international cooperation, in rural infrastructure, agricultural research and extension services, technology development and plant and livestock gene banks in order to enhance agricultural productive capacity in developing countries, in particular least developed countries
- Correct and prevent trade restrictions and distortions in world agricultural markets, including through the parallel elimination of all forms of agricultural export subsidies and all export measures with equivalent effect, in accordance with the mandate of the Doha Development Round
- Adopt measures to ensure the proper functioning of food commodity markets and their derivatives and facilitate timely access to market information, including on food reserves, in order to help limit extreme food price volatility.

Goal 3: Ensure Healthy Lives and Promote Well-Being for All at All Ages

- By 2030, reduce the global maternal mortality ratio to less than 70 per 100,000 live births
- By 2030, end preventable deaths of newborns and children under 5 years of age, with all countries aiming to reduce neonatal mortality to at least as low as 12 per 1,000 live births and under-5 mortality to at least as low as 25 per 1,000 live births

- By 2030, end the epidemics of AIDS, tuberculosis, malaria and neglected tropical diseases and combat hepatitis, water-borne diseases and other communicable diseases
- By 2030, reduce by one third premature mortality from non-communicable diseases through prevention and treatment and promote mental health and well-being
- Strengthen the prevention and treatment of substance abuse, including narcotic drug abuse and harmful use of alcohol
- By 2020, halve the number of global deaths and injuries from road traffic accidents 3.7 By 2030, ensure universal access to sexual and reproductive health-care services, including for family planning, information and education, and the integration of reproductive health into national strategies and programs
- Achieve universal health coverage, including financial risk protection, access to quality essential health-care services and access to safe, effective, quality and affordable essential medicines and vaccines for all
- By 2030, substantially reduce the number of deaths and illnesses from hazardous chemicals and air, water and soil pollution and contamination
- Strengthen the implementation of the World Health Organization Framework Convention on Tobacco Control in all countries, as appropriate
- Support the research and development of vaccines and medicines for the communicable and non-communicable diseases that primarily affect developing countries, provide access to affordable essential medicines and vaccines, in accordance with the Doha Declaration on the TRIPS Agreement and Public Health, which affirms the right of developing countries to use to the full the provisions in the Agreement on Trade Related Aspects of Intellectual Property Rights regarding flexibilities to protect public health, and, in particular, provide access to medicines for all
- Substantially increase health financing and the recruitment, development, training and retention of the health workforce in developing countries, especially in least developed countries and small island developing States
- Strengthen the capacity of all countries, in particular developing countries, for early warning, risk reduction and management of national and global health risks.

Goal 4: Ensure Inclusive and Quality Education for All and Promote Lifelong Learning

- By 2030, ensure that all girls and boys complete free, equitable and quality primary and secondary education leading to relevant and Goal-4 effective learning outcomes
- By 2030, ensure that all girls and boys have access to quality early childhood development, care and preprimary education so that they are ready for primary education
- By 2030, ensure equal access for all women and men to affordable and quality technical, vocational and tertiary education, including university
- By 2030, substantially increase the number of youth and adults who have relevant skills, including technical and vocational skills, for employment, decent jobs and entrepreneurship

- By 2030, eliminate gender disparities in education and ensure equal access to all levels of education and vocational training for the vulnerable, including persons with disabilities, indigenous peoples and children in vulnerable situations
- By 2030, ensure that all youth and a substantial proportion of adults, both men and women, achieve literacy and numeracy
- By 2030, ensure that all learners acquire the knowledge and skills needed to promote sustainable development, including, among others, through education for sustainable development and sustainable lifestyles, human rights, gender equality, promotion of a culture of peace and non-violence, global citizenship and appreciation of cultural diversity and of culture's contribution to sustainable development
- Build and upgrade education facilities that are child, disability and gender sensitive and provide safe, nonviolent, inclusive and effective learning environments for all
- By 2020, substantially expand globally the number of scholarships available to developing countries, in particular least developed countries, small island developing States and African countries, for enrolment in higher education, including vocational training and information and communications technology, technical, engineering and scientific programs, in developed countries and other developing countries
- By 2030, substantially increase the supply of qualified teachers, including through international cooperation for teacher training in developing countries, especially least developed countries and small island developing states.

Goal 5: Achieve Gender Equality and Empower All Women and Girls

- End all forms of discrimination against all women and girls everywhere
- Eliminate all forms of violence against all women and girls in the public and private spheres, including trafficking and sexual and other types of exploitation
- Eliminate all harmful practices, such as child, early and forced marriage and female genital mutilation
- Recognize and value unpaid care and domestic work through the provision of public services, infrastructure and social protection policies and the promotion of shared responsibility within the household and the family as nationally appropriate
- Ensure women's full and effective participation and equal opportunities for leadership at all levels of decision making in political, economic and public life
- Ensure universal access to sexual and reproductive health and reproductive rights as agreed in accordance with the Program of Action of the International Conference on Population and Development and the Beijing Platform for Action and the outcome documents of their review conferences
- Undertake reforms to give women equal rights to economic resources, as well as access to ownership and control over land and other forms of property, financial services, inheritance and natural resources, in accordance with national laws
- Enhance the use of enabling technology, in particular information and communications technology, to promote the empowerment of women
- Adopt and strengthen sound policies and enforceable legislation for the promotion of gender equality and the empowerment of all women and girls at all levels.

Goal 6: Ensure Availability and Sustainable Management of Water and Sanitation for All

- By 2030, achieve universal and equitable access to safe and affordable drinking water for all
- By 2030, achieve access to adequate and equitable sanitation and hygiene for all, and end open defecation, paying special attention to the needs of women and girls and those in vulnerable situations
- By 2030, improve water quality by reducing pollution, eliminating dumping and minimizing release of hazardous chemicals and materials, halving the proportion of untreated wastewater, and increasing recycling and safe reuse by x% globally
- By 2030, substantially increase water-use efficiency across all sectors and ensure sustainable withdrawals and supply of freshwater to address water scarcity, and substantially reduce the number of people suffering from water scarcity
- By 2030 implement integrated water resources management at all levels, including through trans boundary cooperation as appropriate
- By 2020 protect and restore water-related ecosystems, including mountains, forests, wetlands, rivers, aquifers and lakes
- By 2030, expand international cooperation and capacity-building support to developing countries in water and sanitation related activities and programs, including water harvesting, desalination, water efficiency, wastewater treatment, recycling and reuse technologies
- Support and strengthen the participation of local communities for improving water and sanitation management.

Goal 7: Ensure Access to Affordable, Reliable, Sustainable, and Modern Energy for All

- By 2030 ensure universal access to affordable, reliable, and modern energy services
- Increase substantially the share of renewable energy in the global energy mix by 2030
- Double the global rate of improvement in energy efficiency by 2030
- By 2030 enhance international cooperation to facilitate access to clean energy research and technologies, including renewable energy, energy efficiency, and advanced and cleaner fossil fuel technologies, and promote investment in energy infrastructure and clean energy technologies
- By 2030 expand infrastructure and upgrade technology for supplying modern and sustainable energy services for all in developing countries, particularly LDCs and SIDS.

Goal 8: Promote Sustained, Inclusive and Sustainable Economic Growth, Full and Productive Employment and Decent Work for All

- Sustain per capita economic growth in accordance with national circumstances, and in particular at least 7% per annum GDP growth in the least-developed countries
- Achieve higher levels of productivity of economies through diversification, technological upgrading and innovation, including through a focus on high value added and labour-intensive sectors
- Promote development-oriented policies that support productive activities, decent job creation, entrepreneurship, creativity and innovation, and encourage formalization and growth of micro-, small- and medium-sized enterprises including through access to financial services
- Improve progressively through 2030 global resource efficiency in consumption and production, and endeavor to decouple economic growth from environmental degradation in accordance with the 10-year framework of programs on sustainable consumption and production with developed countries taking the lead
- By 2030 achieve full and productive employment and decent work for all women and men, including for young people and persons with disabilities, and equal pay for work of equal value
- By 2020 substantially reduce the proportion of youth not in employment, education or training
- Take immediate and effective measures to secure the prohibition and elimination of the worst forms of child labor, eradicate forced labor, and by 2025 end child labor in all its forms including recruitment and use of child soldiers
- Protect labor rights and promote safe and secure working environments of all workers, including migrant workers, particularly women migrants, and those in precarious employment
- By 2030 devise and implement policies to promote sustainable tourism which creates jobs, promotes local culture and products
- Strengthen the capacity of domestic financial institutions to encourage and to expand access to banking, insurance and financial services for all
- Increase Aid for Trade support for developing countries, particularly LDCs, including through the Enhanced Integrated Framework for LDCs
- By 2020 develop and operationalize a global strategy for youth employment and implement the ILO Global Jobs Pact.

Goal 9: Build Resilient Infrastructure, Promote Inclusive and Sustainable Industrialization and Foster Innovation

- Develop quality, reliable, sustainable and resilient infrastructure, including regional and trans-border infrastructure, to support economic development and human well-being, with a focus on affordable and equitable access for all
- Promote inclusive and sustainable industrialization, and by 2030 raise significantly industry's share of employment and GDP in line with national circumstances, and double its share in LDCs

- Increase the access of small-scale industrial and other enterprises, particularly in developing countries, to financial services including affordable credit and their integration into value chains and markets
- By 2030 upgrade infrastructure and retrofit industries to make them sustainable, with increased resource use efficiency and greater adoption of clean and environmentally sound technologies and industrial processes, all countries taking action in accordance with their respective capabilities
- Enhance scientific research, upgrade the technological capabilities of industrial sectors in all countries, particularly developing countries, including by 2030 encouraging innovation and increasing the number of R&D workers per one million people by x% and public and private R&D spending
- Facilitate sustainable and resilient infrastructure development in developing countries through enhanced financial, technological and technical support to African countries, LDCs, LLDCs and SIDS
- Support domestic technology development, research and innovation in developing countries including by ensuring a conducive policy environment for inter alia industrial diversification and value addition to commodities
- Significantly increase access to ICT and strive to provide universal and affordable access to internet in LDCs by 2020.

Goal 10: Reduce Inequality within and among Countries

- By 2030 progressively achieve and sustain income growth of the bottom 40% of the population at a rate higher than the national average
- By 2030 empower and promote the social, economic and political inclusion of all irrespective of age, sex, disability, race, ethnicity, origin, religion or economic or other status
- Ensure equal opportunity and reduce inequalities of outcome, including through eliminating discriminatory laws, policies and practices and promoting appropriate legislation, policies and actions in this regard
- Adopt policies especially fiscal, wage, and social protection policies and progressively achieve greater equality
- Improve regulation and monitoring of global financial markets and institutions and strengthen implementation of such regulations
- Ensure enhanced representation and voice of developing countries in decision making in global international economic and financial institutions in order to deliver more effective, credible, accountable and legitimate institutions
- Facilitate orderly, safe, regular and responsible migration and mobility of people, including through implementation of planned and well managed migration policies
- Implement the principle of special and differential treatment for developing countries, in particular least developed countries, in accordance with WTO agreements
- Encourage ODA and financial flows, including foreign direct investment, to states where the need is greatest, in particular LDCs, African countries, SIDS, and LLDCs, in accordance with their national plans and programs

- By 2030, reduce to less than 3% the transaction costs of migrant remittances and eliminate remittance corridors with costs higher than 5%.

Goal 11: Make Cities and Human Settlements Inclusive, Safe, Resilient and Sustainable

- By 2030, ensure access for all to adequate, safe and affordable housing and basic services, and upgrade slums
- By 2030, provide access to safe, affordable, accessible and sustainable transport systems for all, improving road safety, notably by expanding public transport, with special attention to the needs of those in vulnerable situations, women, children, persons with disabilities and older persons
- By 2030 enhance inclusive and sustainable urbanization and capacities for participatory, integrated and sustainable human settlement planning and management in all countries
- Strengthen efforts to protect and safeguard the world's cultural and natural heritage
- By 2030 significantly reduce the number of deaths and the number of affected people and decrease by y% the economic losses relative to GDP caused by disasters, including water-related disasters, with the focus on protecting the poor and people in vulnerable situations
- By 2030, reduce the adverse per capita environmental impact of cities, including by paying special attention to air quality, municipal and other waste management
- By 2030, provide universal access to safe, inclusive and accessible, green and public spaces, particularly for women and children, older persons and persons with disabilities
- Support positive economic, social and environmental links between urban, peri-urban and rural areas by strengthening national and regional development planning
- By 2020, increase by x% the number of cities and human settlements adopting and implementing integrated policies and plans towards inclusion, resource efficiency, mitigation and adaptation to climate change, resilience to disasters, develop and implement in line with the forthcoming Hyogo Framework holistic disaster risk management at all levels
- Support least developed countries, including through financial and technical assistance, for sustainable and resilient buildings utilizing local materials.

Goal 12: Ensure Sustainable Consumption and Production Patterns

- Implement the 10-Year Framework of Programs on sustainable consumption and production (10YFP), all countries taking action, with developed countries taking the lead, taking into account the development and capabilities of developing countries
- By 2030 achieve sustainable management and efficient use of natural resources
- By 2030 halve per capita global food waste at the retail and consumer level, and reduce food losses along production and supply chains including post-harvest losses

- By 2020 achieve environmentally sound management of chemicals and all wastes throughout their life cycle in accordance with agreed international frameworks and significantly reduce their release to air, water and soil to minimize their adverse impacts on human health and the environment
- By 2030, substantially reduce waste generation through prevention, reduction, recycling, and reuse
- Encourage companies, especially large and trans-national companies, to adopt sustainable practices and to integrate sustainability information into their reporting cycle
- Promote public procurement practices that are sustainable in accordance with national policies and priorities
- By 2030 ensure that people everywhere have the relevant information and awareness for sustainable development and lifestyles in harmony with nature
- Support developing countries to strengthen their scientific and technological capacities to move towards more sustainable patterns of consumption and production
- Develop and implement tools to monitor sustainable development impacts for sustainable tourism which creates jobs, promotes local culture and products
- Rationalize inefficient fossil fuel subsidies that encourage wasteful consumption by removing market distortions, in accordance with national circumstances, including by restructuring taxation and phasing out those harmful subsidies, where they exist, to reflect their environmental impacts, taking fully into account the specific needs and conditions of developing countries and minimizing the possible adverse impacts on their development in a manner that protects the poor and the affected communities.

Goal 13: Take Urgent Action to Combat Climate Change and Its Impacts*

*Acknowledging that the UNFCCC is the primary international, intergovernmental forum for negotiating the global response to climate change

- Strengthen resilience and adaptive capacity to climate related hazards and natural disasters in all countries
- Integrate climate change measures into national policies, strategies, and planning
- Improve education, awareness raising and human and institutional capacity on climate change mitigation, adaptation, impact reduction, and early warning
- Implement the commitment undertaken by developed country Parties to the UNFCCC to a goal of mobilizing jointly USD100 billion annually by 2020 from all sources to address the needs of developing countries in the context of meaningful mitigation actions and transparency on implementation and fully operationalize the Green Climate Fund through its capitalization as soon as possible
- Promote mechanisms for raising capacities for effective climate change related planning and management, in LDCs, including focusing on women, youth, local and marginalized communities.

Goal 14: Conserve and Sustainably Use the Oceans, Seas and Marine Resources for Sustainable Development

- By 2025, prevent and significantly reduce marine pollution of all kinds, particularly from land-based activities, including marine debris and nutrient pollution
- By 2020, sustainably manage and protect marine and coastal ecosystems to avoid significant adverse impacts, including by strengthening their resilience, and take action for their restoration, to achieve healthy and productive oceans
- Minimize and address the impacts of ocean acidification, including through enhanced scientific cooperation at all levels
- By 2020, effectively regulate harvesting, and end overfishing, illegal, unreported and unregulated (IUU) fishing and destructive fishing practices and implement science-based management plans, to restore fish stocks in the shortest time feasible at least to levels that can produce maximum sustainable yield as determined by their biological characteristics
- By 2020, conserve at least 10 per cent of coastal and marine areas, consistent with national and international law and based on best available scientific information
- By 2020, prohibit certain forms of fisheries subsidies which contribute to overcapacity and overfishing, and eliminate subsidies that contribute to IUU fishing, and refrain from introducing new such subsidies, recognizing that appropriate and effective special and differential treatment for developing and least developed countries should be an integral part of the WTO fisheries subsidies negotiation *
- By 2030 increase the economic benefits to SIDS and LDCs from the sustainable use of marine resources, including through sustainable management of fisheries, aquaculture and tourism
- Increase scientific knowledge, develop research capacities and transfer marine technology taking into account the Intergovernmental Oceanographic Commission Criteria and Guidelines on the Transfer of Marine Technology, in order to improve ocean health and to enhance the contribution of marine biodiversity to the development of developing countries, in particular SIDS and LDCs
- Provide access of small-scale artisanal fishers to marine resources and markets
- Ensure the full implementation of international law, as reflected in UNCLOS for states parties to it, including, where applicable, existing regional and international regimes for the conservation and sustainable use of oceans and their resources by their parties.

Goal 15: Protect, Restore and Promote Sustainable Use of Terrestrial Ecosystems, Sustainably Manage Forests, Combat Desertification, and Halt and Reverse Land Degradation and Halt Biodiversity Loss

- By 2020 ensure conservation, restoration and sustainable use of terrestrial and inland freshwater ecosystems and their services, in particular forests, wetlands, mountains and dry lands, in line with obligations under international agreements

- By 2020, promote the implementation of sustainable management of all types of forests, halt deforestation, restore degraded forests, and increase afforestation and reforestation by x% globally
- By 2020, combat desertification, and restore degraded land and soil, including land affected by desertification, drought and floods, and strive to achieve a land-degradation neutral world
- By 2030 ensure the conservation of mountain ecosystems, including their biodiversity, to enhance their capacity to provide benefits which are essential for sustainable development
- Take urgent and significant action to reduce degradation of natural habitat, halt the loss of biodiversity, and by 2020 protect and prevent the extinction of threatened species
- Ensure fair and equitable sharing of the benefits arising from the utilization of genetic resources, and promote appropriate access to genetic resources
- Take urgent action to end poaching and trafficking of protected species of flora and fauna, and address both demand and supply of illegal wildlife products
- By 2020 introduce measures to prevent the introduction and significantly reduce the impact of invasive alien species on land and water ecosystems, and control or eradicate the priority species
- By 2020, integrate ecosystems and biodiversity values into national and local planning, development processes and poverty reduction strategies, and accounts
- Mobilize and significantly increase from all sources financial resources to conserve and sustainably use biodiversity and ecosystems
- Mobilize significantly resources from all sources and at all levels to finance sustainable forest management, and provide adequate incentives to developing countries to advance sustainable forest management, including for conservation and reforestation
- Enhance global support to efforts to combat poaching and trafficking of protected species, including by increasing the capacity of local communities to pursue sustainable livelihood opportunities.

Goal 16: Promote Peaceful and Inclusive Societies for Sustainable Development, Provide Access to Justice for All and Build Effective, Accountable and Inclusive Institutions at All Levels

- Significantly reduce all forms of violence and related death rates everywhere
- End abuse, exploitation, trafficking and all forms of violence and torture against children
- Promote the rule of law at the national and international levels, and ensure equal access to justice for all
- By 2030 significantly reduce illicit financial and arms flows, strengthen recovery and return of stolen assets, and combat all forms of organized crime
- Substantially reduce corruption and bribery in all its forms
- Develop effective, accountable and transparent institutions at all levels

- Ensure responsive, inclusive, participatory and representative decision-making at all levels
- Broaden and strengthen the participation of developing countries in the institutions of global governance
- By 2030 provide legal identity for all including birth registration
- Ensure public access to information and protect fundamental freedoms, in accordance with national legislation and international agreements
- Strengthen relevant national institutions, including through international cooperation, for building capacities at all levels, in particular in developing countries, for preventing violence and combating terrorism and crime
- Promote and enforce non-discriminatory laws and policies for sustainable development.

Goal 17: Strengthen the Means of Implementation and Revitalize the Global Partnership for Sustainable Development Finance

- Strengthen domestic resource mobilization, including through international support to developing countries to improve domestic capacity for tax and other revenue collection
- Developed countries to implement fully their ODA commitments, including to provide 0.7% of GNI in ODA to developing countries of which 0.15-0.20% to least-developed countries
- Mobilize additional financial resources for developing countries from multiple sources
- Assist developing countries in attaining long-term debt sustainability through coordinated policies aimed at fostering debt financing, debt relief and debt restructuring, as appropriate, and address the external debt of highly indebted poor countries (HIPC) to reduce debt distress
- Adopt and implement investment promotion regimes for LDCs.

Technology

- Enhance North-South, South-South and triangular regional and international cooperation on and access to science, technology and innovation, and enhance knowledge sharing on mutually agreed terms, including through improved coordination among existing mechanisms, particularly at UN level, and through a global technology facilitation mechanism when agreed
- Promote development, transfer, dissemination and diffusion of environmentally sound technologies to developing countries on favourable terms, including on concessional and preferential terms, as mutually agreed
- Fully operationalize the Technology Bank and STI (Science, Technology and Innovation) capacity building mechanism for LDCs by 2017, and enhance the use of enabling technologies in particular ICT.

Capacity Building

- Enhance international support for implementing effective and targeted capacity building in developing countries to support national plans to implement all sustainable development goals, including through North-South, South-South, and triangular cooperation.

Trade

- Promote a universal, rules-based, open, non-discriminatory and equitable multilateral trading system under the WTO including through the conclusion of negotiations within its Doha Development Agenda
- Increase significantly the exports of developing countries, in particular with a view to doubling the LDC share of global exports by 2020
- Realize timely implementation of duty-free, quota-free market access on a lasting basis for all least developed countries consistent with WTO decisions, including through ensuring that preferential rules of origin applicable to imports from LDCs are transparent and simple, and contribute to facilitating market access.

Systemic Issues

Policy and Institutional Coherence

- Enhance global macroeconomic stability including through policy coordination and policy coherence
- Enhance policy coherence for sustainable development
- Respect each country's policy space and leadership to establish and implement policies for poverty eradication and sustainable development.

Multi-Stakeholder Partnerships

- Enhance the global partnership for sustainable development complemented by multi-stakeholder partnerships that mobilize and share knowledge, expertise, technologies and financial resources to support the achievement of sustainable development goals in all countries, particularly developing countries
- Encourage and promote effective public, public-private, and civil society partnerships, building on the experience and resourcing strategies of partnerships.

Data, Monitoring and Accountability

- By 2020, enhance capacity building support to developing countries, including for LDCs and SIDS, to increase significantly the availability of high-quality, timely and reliable data disaggregated by income, gender, age, race, ethnicity, migratory status, disability, geographic location and other characteristics relevant in national contexts
- By 2030, build on existing initiatives to develop measurements of progress on sustainable development that complement GDP, and support statistical capacity building in developing countries.

Appendix B

Declaration of commitment of Port of Spain: securing our citizens' future by promoting human prosperity, energy security and environmental sustainability. Port of Spain: Summit of the Americas (Available at: www.oas.org/psf/docs/Declaration; accessed 01/24/2014).

We, the Heads of Government of the Caribbean Community (CARICOM), meeting at the Crowne Plaza Hotel, Port-of-Spain, Trinidad and Tobago on 15 September 2007 on the occasion of a special Regional Summit on Chronic Non-Communicable Diseases (NCDs); conscious of the collective actions, which have in the past fuelled regional integration, the goal of which is to enhance the well-being of the citizens of our countries;

Recalling the Nassau Declaration (2001), that "the health of the Region is the wealth of Region," which underscored the importance of health to development;

Inspired by the successes of our joint and several efforts that resulted in the Caribbean being the first Region in the world to eradicate poliomyelitis and measles;

Affirming the main recommendations of the Caribbean Commission on Health and Development which included strategies to prevent and control heart disease, stroke, diabetes, hypertension, obesity and cancer in the Region by addressing their causal risk factors of unhealthy diets, physical inactivity, tobacco use and alcohol abuse and strengthening our health services;

Impelled by a determination to reduce the suffering and burdens caused by NCDs on the citizens of our Region which is the one worst affected in the Americas;

Fully convinced that the burdens of NCDs can be reduced by comprehensive and integrated preventive and control strategies at the individual, family, community, national and regional levels and through collaborative programs, partnerships and policies supported by governments, private sectors, NGOs and our other social, regional and international partners;

Declare –

- Our full support for the initiatives and mechanisms aimed at strengthening regional health institutions, to provide critical leadership required for implementing our agreed strategies for the reduction of the burden of Chronic, Non-Communicable Diseases as a central priority of the Caribbean Cooperation in Health Initiative Phase III (CCH III), being coordinated by the CARICOM Secretariat, with able support from the Pan American Health Organization/World Health Organization (PAHO/WHO) and other relevant partners;

- That we strongly encourage the establishment of National Commissions on NCDs or analogous bodies to plan and coordinate the comprehensive prevention and control of chronic NCDs;
- Our commitment to pursue immediately a legislative agenda for passage of the legal provisions related to the International Framework Convention on Tobacco Control; urge its immediate ratification in all States which have not already done so and support the immediate enactment of legislation to limit or eliminate smoking in public places, ban the sale, advertising and promotion of tobacco products to children, insist on effective warning labels and introduce such fiscal measures as will reduce accessibility of tobacco;
- That public revenue derived from tobacco, alcohol or other such products should be employed, inter alia for preventing chronic NCDs, promoting health and supporting the work of the Commissions;
- That our Ministries of Health, in collaboration with other sectors, will establish by mid-2008 comprehensive plans for the screening and management of chronic diseases and risk factors so that by 2012, 80% of people with NCDs would receive quality care and have access to preventive education based on regional guidelines;
- That we will mandate the re-introduction of physical education in our schools where necessary, provide incentives and resources to effect this policy and ensure that our education sectors promote programs aimed at providing healthy school meals and promoting healthy eating;
- Our endorsement of the efforts of the Caribbean Food and Nutrition Institute (CFNI), Caribbean Agricultural Research and Development Institute (CARDI) and the regional inter-governmental agencies to enhance food security and our strong support for the elimination of trans-fats from the diet of our citizens, using the CFNI as a focal point for providing guidance and public education designed toward this end;
- Our support for the efforts of the Caribbean Regional Negotiating Machinery (CRNM) to pursue fair trade policies in all international trade negotiations thereby promoting greater use of indigenous agricultural products and foods by our populations and reducing the negative effects of globalization on our food supply;
- Our support for mandating the labeling of foods or such measures as are necessary to indicate their nutritional content through the establishment of the appropriate regional capability;
- That we will promote policies and actions aimed at increasing physical activity in the entire population, e.g., at work sites, through sport, especially mass activities, as vehicles for improving the health of the population and conflict resolution and in this context we commit to increasing adequate public facilities such as parks and other recreational spaces to encourage physical activity by the widest cross-section of our citizens;
- Our commitment to take account of the gender dimension in all our programs aimed at the prevention and control of NCDs;
- That we will provide incentives for comprehensive public education programs in support of wellness, healthy life-style changes, improved self-management of NCDs and embrace the role of the media as a responsible partner in all our efforts to prevent and control NCDs;

- That we will establish, as a matter of urgency, the programs necessary for research and surveillance of the risk factors for NCDs with the support of our Universities and the Caribbean Epidemiology Centre/Pan American Health Organization (CAREC/PAHO);

Our continuing support for CARICOM and PAHO as the joint Secretariat for the Caribbean Cooperation in Health (CCH) Initiative to be the entity responsible for revision of the regional plan for the prevention and control of NCDs, and the monitoring and evaluation of this Declaration.

We hereby declare the second Saturday in September "Caribbean Wellness Day," in commemoration of this landmark Summit.

Appendix C

Monitoring compliance with high-level commitments in health: the case of the CARICOM Summit on chronic non-communicable diseases (Samuels et al., 2014)

Appendix C. Revised grid for the reporting of countries' compliance with the 15 mandates of the declaration of Port of Spain, 2010

Mandate number	NCD progress indicator	ANG	ANT	BAH	BAR	BEL	BER	BVI	CAY	DCM	GRE	GUY	HAI	JAM	MON	SKN	STL	SUR	SVG	TCI	TRT
Commitment																					
1,14	NCD plan	X	X	±	√	±	√	√	√	√	√	√	x	√	–	√	√	±	±	X	√
4	NCD budget	X	±	X	√	X	X	X	√	±	X	±	x	X	–	X	√	X	X	X	√
2	NCD Summit convened	X	√	X	√	X	√	√	X	√	±	√	x	√	–	X	√	√	X	X	√

Appendix C. (Continued)

Mandate number	NCD progress indicator	ANG	ANT	BAH	BAR	BEL	BER	BVI	CAY	DOM	GRE	GUY	HAI	JAM	MON	SKN	STL	SUR	SVG	TCI	TRT
2	Multisectoral NCD commission appointed and functional	X	X	X	√	±	√	√	X	±	√	√	x	±	–	X	√	±	X	X	√
12	NCD communications plan	X	X	±	±	X	√	X	√	±	±	√	x	±	–	X	±	±	X	X	√
Tobacco																					
3	FCTC ratified	*	√	√	√	√	*	*	√	√	√	√	x	√	*	√	√	√	√	*	√
3	Tobacco taxes >50% sale price	X	X	X	√	X	–	X	±	X		√	x	√	–	±	X	√	X	X	X
3	Smoke-free indoor public places	X	√	X	√	±	√	√	√	±	√	√	x	±	–	X	√	±	X	X	√
3	Advertising, promotion and sponsorship bans	X	X	X	√	X	√	√	√	X	X	±	x	√	–	X	X	±	X	X	√
Nutrition																					
7	Multisector food and nutrition plan implemented	√	√	√	√	±	X	√	X	√	√	√	x	√	√	√	X	X	√	±	±
7	Trans-fat-free food supply	–	–	–	–	X	–	–	X	X	–	–	–	±	–	–	X	X	X	X	X

Mandate number	NCD progress indicator	ANG	ANT	BAH	BAR	BEL	BER	BVI	CAY	DOM	GRE	GUY	HAI	JAM	MON	SKN	STL	SUR	SVG	TCI	TRT
7	Policy and standards promoting healthy eating in schools implemented	–	√	–	√	±	√	X	±	±	–	±	–	√	–	±	X	X	X	X	±
8	Trade agreements used to meet national food security & health goals	–	–	–	–	X	–	–	X	–	–	±	–	X	–	–	X	X	X	X	√
9	Mandatory labelling of packaged foods for nutrition content	–	X	–	–	X	±	–	±	±	–	±	–	X	–	–	X	±	X	X	X
Physical activity																					
6	Mandatory physical activity in all grades in schools	–	–	–	√	√	±	±	√	√	–	±	–	±	–	–	X	X	X	√	√
10	Mandatory provision in new housing developments	–	–	–	√	√	–	–	X	X	–	X	–	x	–	–	X	X	X	X	X
10	Ongoing, mass physical activity or new public physical activity spaces	X	√	√	√	√	√	X	√	√	√	√	–	√	–	√	√	√	√	X	√
Education/health promotion																					
15	Multisectoral, multifocal CWD celebrations	√	√	√	√	√	√	√	√	√	√	√	x	√	√	√	√	√	√	√	√

Appendix C. (Continued)

Mandate number	NCD progress indicator	ANG	ANT	BAH	BAR	BEL	BER	BVI	CAY	DOM	GRE	GUY	HAI	JAM	MON	SKN	STL	SUR	SVG	TCI	TRT
10	≥ 50% of public and private institutions with physical activity and healthy eating programmes	–	X	–	–	X	–	X	X	X	–	±	–	–	–	–	±	X	X	X	±
12	Media broadcasts on NCD control (risk factors, treatment) >30 days a year	–	√	–	√	X	√	X	±	±	–	√	–	√	–	√	±	X	X	X	√
Surveillance																					
	STEPS or equivalent survey	X	X	√	√	√	±	√	±	√	√	±	x	√	–	√	±	±	X	±	√
	Minimum data set reporting	X	X	√	√	√	√	√	√	√	±	±	x	√	X	√	√	√	√	X	√
11, 13, 14	Global Youth Tobacco Survey	X	√	√	√	√	X	√	±	√	√	√	√	√	–	±	√	√	√	X	√
	Global School Health Survey	√	√	√	±	±	–	√	±	√	√	√	x	√	–	±	√	√	√	X	√
Treatment																					
5	Chronic care model/NCD treatment protocols in ≥ 50% PHC facilities	X	√	√	±	±	±	±	±	X	±	±	x	√	–	X	√	X	X	X	√

Mandate number	NCD progress indicator	ANG	ANT	BAH	BAR	BEL	BER	BVI	CAY	DOM	GRE	GUY	HAI	JAM	MON	SKN	STL	SUR	SVG	TCI	TRT
5	Quality-of-care cardiovascular disease or diabetes demonstration project	=	–	√	√	±	±	±	√	X	√	√	±	√	–	±	√	√	X	X	√

ANG, Anguilla; ANT, Antigua and Barbuda; BAH, Bahamas; BAR, Barbados; BEL, Belize; BER, Bermuda; BVI, British Virgin Islands; CAY, Cayman Islands; CWD, Caribbean Wellness Day; DOM, Dominica; FCTC, Framework Convention on Tobacco Control; GRE, Grenada; GUY, Guyana; HAI, Haiti; JAM, Jamaica; MON, Montserrat; NCD, noncommunicable disease; PHC, primary health care; SKN, Saint Kitts and Nevis; STEPS, STEPwise approach to surveillance; STL, Saint Lucia; SVG, Saint Vincent and the Grenadines; SUR, Suriname; TCI, Turks and Caicos; TRT, Trinidad and Tobago.

Note: The symbols are to be interpreted as follows: √: accomplished; ± : in process/partially implemented; X: not accomplished; *: not applicable; –: missing information.

Index

access, xvi, 26, 37, 41, 44, 45, 46, 48, 52, 53, 54, 56, 57, 66, 67, 68, 80, 85, 89, 90, 106, 111, 113, 150, 153, 154, 155, 156, 157, 158, 159, 160, 162, 163, 164, 165, 168
accessibility, 24, 49, 119, 137, 168
accountability, 60, 62, 140
acquired immunodeficiency syndrome, 62
activity level, xii, xvi, 99, 102, 121
adaptation, 104, 135, 140, 147, 154, 160, 161
adiposity, 118, 137
adjustment, 110
adolescents, 75, 82, 83, 85, 98, 144
adulthood, 10
adults, 74, 75, 76, 82, 83, 84, 95, 99, 100, 101, 107, 118, 132, 136, 140, 141, 144, 146, 149, 150, 155, 156
advertisements, 85
advocacy, xvi, 58, 59, 63, 65, 69
Afghanistan, 11
Africa, xv, 3, 11, 12, 13, 14, 15, 17, 18, 19, 21, 22, 29, 44, 46, 47, 75, 76, 78, 98, 104, 106, 131, 132, 135, 136, 141, 143, 144, 147, 151
age, vii, xv, 9, 19, 23, 25, 33, 37, 76, 88, 100, 110, 117, 123, 133, 135, 148, 154, 159, 165
aging population, xv, 29
agricultural export subsidies, 154
agricultural market, 154
AIDS, xi, 62, 155
air pollutants, 107
air quality, 110, 150, 160
airways, 9
Albania, 11
albumin, 45
alcohol abuse, 73, 124, 167
alcohol consumption, 26, 69
alcohol use, 25
aldosterone, 139
Algeria, 11
alien species, 163
American Heart Association, xi, 88, 97
American Samoa, 11
amino acids, 83
amputation, 139
Angola, 11, 76
antihypertensive drugs, 46, 127
aquaculture, 162
aquifers, 157
Argentina, 11, 81, 97, 98, 102, 143
Armenia, 11
aromatic hydrocarbons, xii
arthritis, 134
Asia, 21, 22, 46, 106, 135, 140, 144, 145, 147, 149
assessment, 138, 140, 142, 147, 149
assets, 23, 163
asthma, 9, 25, 110, 142
athletes, 83
atmosphere, 103, 104, 108
atoms, 93
attachment, 146
attitudes, 132
Austria, 11
authorities, 59, 81
autonomy, 151
avoidance, 95
awareness, 3, 66, 67, 68, 69, 78, 81, 86, 88, 103, 121, 122, 126, 161
Azerbaijan, 11

B

Bahrain, 11, 81
ban, 168
Bangladesh, 11, 35, 36
banking, 158
banks, 154
Barbados, 11, 35, 62, 123, 175

barriers, 44, 47, 62, 84, 138
base, 47
basic services, 153, 160
behavioral change, 44
behaviors, 52, 57, 122, 145
Beijing, 156
Belarus, 11
Belgium, 11
benefits, 21, 33, 74, 82, 99, 100, 121, 147, 154, 162, 163
benign, 7
benign tumors, 7
beverages, vii, xi, xii, 24, 57, 69, 80, 82, 83, 88, 89, 90, 92, 97, 133, 135, 138, 140, 143, 144, 146, 148, 149
Bhutan, 11, 45, 46
bilateral, 55
bile, 93
bile acids, 93
biodiversity, 162, 163
birth rate, 20, 23
birth weight, 25
births, 154
black women, 142
bladder cancer, 109
bleeding, 6
blindness, 122
blood, 6, 7, 10, 21, 25, 45, 75, 77, 78, 82, 83, 93, 95, 96, 97, 109, 118, 125, 126, 127, 139, 144
blood clot, 6
blood pressure, 21, 25, 75, 77, 78, 82, 96, 97, 125, 127, 139, 144
blood stream, 93
blood vessels, 6, 7, 109
body mass index (BMI) , xi, 21, 73, 97, 101, 113
body weight, 97, 139
Bolivia, 11
bone, 7, 99
bone marrow, 7
Bosnia, 11
Botswana, 11, 76
bowel, 107
brain, 6, 7, 93, 119
brain drain, 119
Brazil, 11, 17, 19, 28, 33, 49, 81, 104, 120, 135, 142, 146
breathlessness, 9
bronchitis, 9
building blocks, 41, 150
Bulgaria, 11
buns, 81
Burkina Faso, 11, 76, 148
Burundi, 11, 76

C

CAD, 133
caffeine, 83, 149
calcium, 127
call centers, 24
caloric intake, 21
calorie, 84, 89
Cambodia, 11
Cameroon, viii, x, xvii, 11, 76, 98, 117, 118, 119, 120, 123, 136, 137, 147, 148
campaigns, xvi, 58, 60, 63, 69, 81, 86
cancer, x, xii, 6, 7, 17, 25, 30,33, 34, 35, 37, 45, 47, 54, 74, 80, 86, 98, 107, 108, 109, 113, 118, 125, 131, 138, 140, 142, 143, 146, 147, 151, 167
  benign versus malignant, ix, 8
  deaths, 20, 76
  definition, 83
  origin, ix, 8
  types, vii, ix, 7, 78
cancer death, 17
capacity building, 55, 164, 165
capital accumulation, 31
carbohydrates, 9, 28, 29
carbon, 92, 93, 104, 111, 113
carbon atoms, 93
carbon emissions, 104
carcinogen, 109
cardiomyopathy, 110, 149
cardiovascular disease (CVD), x, xi, 6, 25, 30, 32, 81, 109, 117, 120, 125, 132, 133, 137, 143, 144, 150, 175
  deaths, 20, 76
  definition, 83
cardiovascular morbidity, 141
cardiovascular risk, 141, 149
care model, ix, xi, 43, 51, 129, 136, 141, 144, 145, 174
caregivers, 85
Caribbean, xi, xv, 3, 11, 12, 13, 14, 15, 18, 19, 21, 61, 62, 123, 124, 132, 133, 134, 135, 137, 139, 140, 144, 167, 168, 169, 175
Caribbean countries, 123
cartilage, 7
case studies, 138
case study, 21, 132, 139
catecholamines, 139
category a, 86, 127
CDC, xi, 66, 83, 88, 90, 102, 135
Central African Republic, 12, 76, 117
Central Asia, 11, 12, 13, 14, 15
cerebrovascular disease, 6, 109
cervical cancer, 48, 123

Chad, 12, 76, 117
Chagas disease, 110
challenges, xv, 5, 41, 45, 46, 49, 52, 65, 105, 132, 136, 137, 141, 146
Chamber of Commerce, 34, 148
cheese, 74, 81
chemical, 109
chemical reactions, 109
chemicals, xvi, 107, 108, 113, 155, 157, 161
chemotherapy, 47
CHF, xi, 120
child labor, 158
childhood, 9, 10, 25, 75, 155
Chile, 12, 28, 81, 131
China, 12, 13, 15, 17, 19, 21, 29, 33, 140, 144
cholesterol, vii, 21, 45, 74, 82, 83, 86, 93, 94, 95, 96, 97, 102, 123, 139, 148, 149
chronic disease(s), ix, xi, xvii, 3, 5, 17, 19, 23, 24, 25, 26, 28, 29, 30, 31, 32, 33, 34, 35, 36, 43, 44, 45, 46, 47, 48, 51, 52, 53, 55, 58, 60, 61, 62, 63, 65, 66, 67, 73, 74, 82, 98, 102, 103, 106, 111, 113, 117, 118, 120, 123, 124, 125, 126, 129, 130, 133, 134, 135, 137, 140, 141, 143, 144, 147, 148, 150, 151, 168
  definition, 83
  mortality, 18, 138
  poverty-chronic disease relationship, ix, 26
  prevalence, 135, 140, 144, 146
  risk factors, vii, 25
chronic illness, 133, 136, 149
chronic kidney disease (CKD), xi, 37, 41
chronic obstructive pulmonary disease, 9, 110
chronic respiratory disease, xi, 9
  definition, 83
  symptoms, 138
cirrhosis, 6
clean energy, 157
climate change, ix, x, xvi, xvii, 3, 103, 104, 105, 106, 107, 108, 109, 110, 111, 112, 113, 132, 136, 137, 140, 145, 149, 150, 154, 160, 161
  human health, 135, 147
climate extremes, 109
CO_2, x, 103, 104, 105
coastal ecosystems, 162
coffee, 83, 88, 89
coherence, 57, 58, 86, 165
collaboration, 49, 60, 67, 68, 69, 78, 80, 81, 122, 124, 168
Colombia, 12
colon cancer, 6, 98
commodity markets, 154
common symptoms, 9
communication, 43, 44, 84
community support, xi, 43, 66, 134
comparative analysis, 147
complications, xvi, 35, 36, 38, 51, 122, 127, 135
conceptualization, 50
conflict resolution, 168
congenital heart disease, 6, 109
Congo, 12, 76, 117
consumer education, 78, 88, 102
consumer markets, 20
consumers, 43, 79, 80, 81, 82, 91, 122
consumption, vii, 24, 28, 29, 56, 59, 73, 75, 76, 80, 81, 82, 83, 84, 85, 86, 88, 90, 95, 96, 97, 102, 111, 126, 132, 135, 136, 138, 141, 143, 145, 149, 158, 160, 161
consumption patterns, 24, 28, 59
contamination, 108, 155
controlled trials, 86, 139
cooking, 67, 79, 87
cooperation, 56, 57, 153, 154, 156, 157, 162, 164, 165
coordination, 55, 68, 164, 165
COPD, xi, 9, 35
copper, 49
coronary artery disease, 145
coronary heart disease, 6, 22, 78, 109, 138
correlations, xvi, 51, 54
corruption, 163
cost, vii, xvi, 5, 30, 31, 33, 34, 35, 36, 37, 38, 43, 44, 46, 47, 49, 50, 53, 56, 57, 58, 61, 75, 77, 100, 102, 104, 105, 119, 121, 126, 127, 131, 132, 135, 137, 140, 145, 149
Costa Rica, 12, 92
counseling, 86, 96, 125
creatinine, 45
Croatia, 12
cross-sectional study, 137
Cuba, 12, 49
cultural norms, 59
culture, 24, 143, 156, 158, 161
cure, 43
CVD, xi, xv, xvi, xvii, 6, 16, 18, 19, 21, 30, 32, 33, 35, 38, 68, 74, 75, 76, 78, 80, 82, 102, 107, 109, 110, 113, 117, 118, 119, 123
Cyprus, 12
Czech Republic, 12, 142

D

data collection, 47, 69
data set, 174
death rate, xv, 19, 20, 23, 95, 123, 163

deaths, vii, ix, xv, 17, 18, 19, 20, 28, 29, 30, 33, 60, 62, 75, 76, 82, 94, 98, 106, 107, 109, 117, 119, 123, 154, 155, 160
deforestation, 163
degradation, 163
dehydration, 111
demographic transition, 28
demonstrations, 67
Denmark, 12
Department of Education, 121
deposits, 6
depression, 33, 68
depressive symptoms, 101
deprivation, 26
depth, 73
derivatives, 154
detection, 44, 68, 69
Determinants of chronic disease
  determinants of chronic disease
    urbanization, 20, 22, 25, 131, 132, 135, 148, 149
  globalization, 24, 25, 29, 136, 137, 151
  population aging, 23, 25
developed countries, xv, xvi, 19, 22, 24, 29, 31, 37, 38, 46, 47, 51, 54, 65, 106, 108, 109, 113, 153, 154, 155, 156, 158, 159, 160, 162, 164, 165
developing countries, vii, xv, xvi, xvii, 3, 5, 11, 17, 19, 20, 21, 22, 23, 24, 28, 29, 30, 31, 33, 35, 36, 37, 38, 41, 43, 44, 45, 46, 47, 49, 50, 52, 54, 55, 56, 57, 58, 75, 79, 80, 82, 102, 103, 104, 106, 109, 110, 111, 113, 118, 119, 120, 121, 125, 129, 130, 132, 133, 134, 137, 138, 140, 144, 147, 153, 154, 155, 156, 157, 158, 159, 160, 161, 162, 163, 164, 165
  classification, 15, 89
  low-income, 15, 16, 76
developing economies, 16
development assistance, 56
development policy, 57
diabetes, vii, viii, ix, x, xi, xii, xv, xvi, xvii, 3, 6, 9, 10, 16, 17, 18, 19, 21, 25, 29, 30, 31, 33, 35, 36, 38, 44, 46, 51, 60, 62, 66, 67, 74, 75, 80, 82, 83, 88, 90, 98, 100, 102, 107, 110, 111, 112, 113, 117, 118, 119, 120, 121, 122, 123, 125, 126, 127, 131, 132, 134, 135, 137, 139, 140, 141, 143, 144, 146, 147, 149, 151, 167, 175
  definition, 83
  prevalence, 135, 140, 144, 146
  type of, 37, 78
diabetic patients, 36, 118
dialysis, 33, 37, 46, 151
dichotomy, 136
diet, xv, 6, 21, 25, 28, 29, 57, 62, 73, 74, 75, 88, 90, 91, 95, 96, 97, 102, 134, 137, 139, 145, 168
dietary fat, xvii, 21, 28, 29, 129
dietary fiber, 73
dietary intake, xvi, 58, 63, 94, 147
differential treatment, 159, 162
diffusion, 164
direct cost, ix, 34, 35, 36
direct payment, 47
direction and way forward
  sample action plans, viii, 127
directives, 124
disability, 30, 33, 38, 94, 106, 136, 156, 159, 165
disaster, 106, 137, 141, 160
discrimination, 38, 156
disease and climate change
  cancer, x, xii, 6, 7, 17, 25, 30, 37, 80, 107, 108, 131, 138, 140, 142, 143, 146, 147
  diabetes, viii, xii, 9, 17, 18, 25, 30, 32, 36, 66, 67, 80, 88, 90, 110, 119, 127, 131, 132, 134, 135, 136, 139, 140, 143, 144, 145, 146, 149, 151
disease rate, 68
diseases, ix, x, xiii, xv, xvi, xvii, 3, 5, 6, 9, 16, 17, 19, 20, 22, 23, 25, 26, 28, 29, 30, 31, 33, 37, 38, 41, 43, 44, 46, 47, 48, 50, 54, 55, 60, 61, 62, 65, 66, 67, 73, 77, 86, 98, 103, 107, 108, 109, 110, 113, 117, 119, 120, 123, 124, 125, 126, 129, 130, 131, 132, 133, 134, 135, 136, 137, 139, 140, 142, 143, 144, 145, 146, 147, 148, 150, 155, 171
distress, 164
distribution, xvii, 28, 29, 46, 47, 49, 50, 103, 109, 113
diversification, 158, 159
diversity, 156
DNA, xi, 7, 109
doctors, 5
Doha, 154, 155, 165
domestic resources, 57
Dominican Republic, 12, 28
donors, 60, 63
drinking water, 90, 157
drought, 110, 154, 163
drug abuse, 155
drug therapy, 125
drugs, 41, 47, 48, 127, 137
dumping, 157

E

early warning, 155, 161
earthquakes, 149
East Asia, xv, 11, 12, 13, 14, 15, 17, 18, 19, 29, 78, 79, 80, 95

ecology, 67, 107
economic crisis, 62
economic damage, 69
economic development, 20, 24, 28, 48, 67, 138, 149, 158
economic globalisation, 146
economic growth, xvi, 15, 24, 29, 30, 33, 38, 60, 158
economic losses, 33, 160
economic resources, 153, 156
economics, 137, 151
economics and chronic disease
conceptual framework, ix, 31
cost of type 2 diabetes, vii, 36
direct cost, 131, 151
economic burden, vii, 30, 131, 137, 141
global economic burden, vii, 32
health expenditure, 151
intangible cost, xvi, 38
lost economic output, ix, 34
Ecuador, 12, 28, 92, 137
education, 21, 43, 44, 48, 67, 78, 81, 84, 87, 89, 90, 91, 119, 126, 127, 155, 156, 158, 161, 168
educational materials, 88
educators, 5
efforts to prevent chronic disease
Caribbean, xi, xv, 3, 11, 12, 13, 14, 15, 18, 19, 21, 61, 62, 123, 124, 132, 133, 134, 135, 137, 139, 140, 144, 167, 168, 169, 175
declaration of Port-of-Spain, 61
Kenya, 13, 60, 61, 76, 141
egg, 93, 96
Egypt, 12, 17
El Salvador, 12
elderly population, 23, 139
electrolyte, 75
electron, 146
emphysema, 9
employees, 33, 90, 136
employment, 154, 155, 158
empowerment, 51, 65, 156
energy, xii, 29, 73, 82, 83, 85, 88, 91, 95, 97, 100, 113, 118, 132, 137, 157, 167
energy density, 85, 137
energy efficiency, 157
energy expenditure, xii, 100, 118, 132
energy security, 167
engineering, 156
England, 24, 28, 69, 139, 146
entrepreneurship, 155, 158
environmental change, 90, 104
environmental degradation, 158
environmental factors, 25, 104
environmental impact, 160, 161
environmental sustainability, 167
EPA, ix, xi, 93, 109
epidemic, xv, 19, 41, 52, 61, 62, 67, 123, 124, 132, 144
epidemiologic, 134
epidemiology, 3
equal opportunity, 159
equality, 159
Equatorial Guinea, 12, 76, 117
Eritrea, 12, 30, 45, 76
Estonia, 12
ethnic groups, 107
ethnicity, 159, 165
Europe, 11, 12, 13, 14, 15, 18, 21, 24, 36, 44, 78, 97, 150
European Commission, 78, 138
evidence, xvii, 22, 25, 58, 65, 67, 84, 85, 86, 87, 101, 102, 103, 109, 110, 113, 117, 118, 124, 126, 129, 131, 133, 149
evidence-based intervention
Agita São Paulo, 120, 121, 132, 143
Cameroon, viii, x, xvii, 11, 76, 98, 117, 118, 119, 120, 123, 136, 137, 147, 148
mDiabetes, 122, 123
Executive Order, xii, 88, 137
exercise, 96, 98, 121, 122, 141
exercise program, 141
expenditures, 35
expertise, 44, 67, 165
exploitation, 156, 163
exports, 165
exposure, xvi, 6, 21, 24, 61, 69, 85, 107, 108, 109, 110, 111, 113, 132, 133, 138, 153
extinction, 163
extreme cold, xvii, 110, 113
extreme poverty, 56, 153
extreme weather events, 107, 110

F

family life, 137
family members, xvii, 36, 119, 129
family planning, 48, 155
farmers, 154
fasting, 10, 97, 118
fasting glucose, 10, 97
fat, 7, 9, 10, 26, 28, 29, 83, 88, 91, 92, 93, 96, 97, 98, 102, 139, 172
fat intake, 29, 139
fatty acids, ix, xii, 29, 74, 92, 93, 94, 96, 97, 138, 144
Federal Government, 49
feelings, 100

female genital mutilation, 156
fertility, 28
fiber, 28, 95, 96, 97
fibers, 75
Fiji, 12
financial institutions, 158, 159
financial markets, 159
financial resources, 41, 163, 164, 165
Finland, 12, 78, 88, 95
fiscal year, 37
fish, 74, 93, 96, 97, 162
fish oil, 93
fisheries, 162
fishing, 162
fitness, 118
flavor, 75
flexibility, 38
flooding, xvi, 108, 113, 154
floods, xvii, 108, 111, 113, 131, 163
flora, 163
flora and fauna, 163
fluid, 75, 88
fluid balance, 75
food additive, 75
food industry, xvii, 3, 5, 57, 77, 78, 80, 81, 86, 102, 111, 129, 139
food production, 28, 29, 87, 113, 154
food products, 77, 78, 96
food security, 168, 173
force, 81, 111
foreign direct investment, 24, 159
forest management, 163
foundations, 51, 63
framing, 121
France, 12, 88, 92, 138
freshwater, 157, 162
fructose, 83, 144, 148
fruits, 26, 28, 73, 84, 92, 95, 96, 122
funding, 46, 48, 56, 68, 124, 130
funds, 46, 56, 63, 100

G

Gabon, 12, 20, 76, 117
GDP, xi, 30, 31, 33, 35, 36, 46, 49, 50, 56, 104, 117, 119, 151, 158, 160, 165
GDP per capita, 117
gender dimension, 168
gender equality, 156
gender-sensitive, 153
general education, 87
generic drugs, 127
genetic diversity, 154
genetic factors, 25
Georgia, 12
Germany, 12, 17, 30, 104
gestational diabetes, 10, 80, 135
global climate change, 142
global demand, 49
global forces, 111
global warming, 105
globalization, xv, 20, 23, 24, 28, 29, 60, 151, 168
glucose, 10, 25, 45, 86, 118, 126, 132, 148
glucose tolerance, 10
glutamate, 75
glycerol, 92, 93
governance, 57, 86, 143, 164
government expenditure, 46
government policy, 87
government spending, 56
governments, xvi, xvii, 24, 46, 49, 58, 61, 62, 63, 67, 68, 86, 88, 123, 126, 129, 130, 140, 167
Greece, 12
greenhouse, x, 103, 105, 111, 113, 134, 147
greenhouse gas, 103, 111, 113, 134
greenhouse gas(es) (GHG), xii, 103, 111, 113, 134
greenhouse gas emissions, 111
Grenada, 12, 175
gross domestic product, 30, 141
growth, vii, 6, 7, 8, 21, 24, 41, 117, 130, 158, 159
growth rate, 117
Guam, 12
Guatemala, 12, 37
guidance, 168
guidelines, 44, 59, 86, 92, 95, 118, 147, 150, 168
Guinea, 12, 14, 76, 117
Guyana, 12, 175

H

habitat, 163
Haiti, 13, 61, 62, 175
harmony, 161
harvesting, 157, 162
hazards, 161
health care, xvi, xvii, 21, 26, 41, 42, 43, 44, 46, 47, 48, 49, 50, 51, 52, 54, 56, 57, 60, 67, 86, 100, 107, 119, 126, 127, 129, 133, 135, 136, 137, 138, 140, 141, 142, 143, 144, 146, 148, 150, 175
health care costs, 56, 107
health care system, 41, 43, 47, 49, 51, 52
health condition, 100
health education, 50
health effects, 132, 133, 135, 136, 145
health expenditure, 29, 35, 37, 46, 56, 119
health insurance, 121, 133, 139

health problems, ix, 33, 34, 48, 49, 148
health promotion, 43, 48, 50, 61, 65, 66, 69, 81, 132, 138, 147, 173
health risks, 155
health services, 42, 47, 48, 49, 50, 56, 131, 167
health status, 65, 133
healthcare models
chronic care model, xi, 174
expanded chronic care model, xi
healthcare systems, xvii, 120
medicines, 44, 127
primary healthcare, xii, 142
strategies to improve, ix, 53, 130
universal healthcare, xii
health-promoting behaviors, 87
hearing loss, 6
heart attack, 6, 96, 97, 110, 111, 125
heart disease, xi, xii, 23, 25, 33, 60, 62, 74, 75, 94, 95, 96, 97, 109, 120, 122, 146, 167
heart failure, xi, 120
heat stroke, 111
heavy metals, 108
hemodialysis, 37
hepatitis, 155
heredity, 25
heterogeneity, 20
high blood cholesterol, 97
high blood pressure, 25, 77, 79
high fiber foods, 96
higher education, 156
HIPC, 164
HIV, 151
Honduras, 13
Hong Kong, 13
horizontal equity, 135
hormone, 10
hormones, 93
hospital death, 60
household income, 35
Housing and Urban Development, 61
human activity, 103
human body, 75
human health, ix, 103, 104, 106, 139, 145, 161
human resources, 41, 67
human right, 156
humidity, 146
Hungary, 13, 88
hydrogen atoms, 92, 93
hygiene, 157
hyperglycemia, 9, 10
hypertension, viii, xi, 23, 62, 67, 74, 75, 80, 82, 97, 98, 109, 120, 121, 123, 126, 127, 134, 141, 143, 146, 147, 149, 167
hypertriglyceridemia, 82
hypothesis, 108, 134

I

Iceland, 13, 126
IDA, 15
immune system, 7, 109
immunization, 48
immunodeficiency, xi
impact assessment, 59
imports, 165
improvements, xvi, 101, 102
impulses, 75
in utero, 25
incidence, 23, 28, 78, 80, 82, 95, 102, 110, 132, 140, 146
increased access, 82
independence, 50
India, 13, 17, 19, 20, 21, 22, 24, 35, 36, 37, 122, 131, 137, 141, 146
Indians, 122
indigenous peoples, 154, 156
indirect effect, 107, 110
individuals, xvii, 5, 10, 17, 23, 24, 28, 37, 48, 49, 50, 52, 65, 80, 86, 87, 99, 111, 113, 117, 121, 123, 129, 135
Indonesia, 13, 17, 22, 149
industrial revolution, 24, 28, 139
industrial sectors, 159
industrialization, 158
infant mortality, 28
infants, 154
infectious agents, 25
inflammation, 9, 83, 140
information technology, 24
infrastructure, xvi, 46, 48, 50, 106, 111, 113, 154, 156, 157, 158, 159
injections, 10, 45
injuries, 48, 155
instant noodles, 81
institutions, 5, 41, 57, 59, 84, 126, 159, 163, 164, 167, 174
insulin, ix, 10, 8, 127, 133, 144, 145, 148
insulin resistance, 83, 144, 148
insulin signaling, 83
integration, 24, 50, 68, 132, 155, 159
interactions and partnerships for prevention
non-governmental organizations, xii
interest groups, 60
International Energy Agency, 103
international law, 162
international trade, 24, 168

intervention, xvi, 58, 59, 63, 66, 68, 90, 100, 102, 121, 122, 126, 145, 151
investment(s), 24, 47, 48, 56, 57, 58, 68, 150, 153, 154, 157, 164
Iran, xvi, 13, 98, 102
Iraq, 13
Ireland, 13, 95
ischaemic heart disease, 139
Islam, 35, 36, 140
Israel, 13
Italy, 13

J

Jamaica, viii, 13, 20, 36, 119, 123, 124, 133, 134, 139, 149, 175
Japan, 13, 17, 37, 140, 149
Java, 149
job creation, 158
Jordan, 13, 51, 137

K

Kazakhstan, 13
Kenya, 13, 60, 61, 76, 141
ketones, 45
kidney, vii, xi, 37, 41, 122, 136, 141
kidney failure, 122
Korea, 13
Kosovo, 13
Kuwait, 13, 81, 142

L

labeling, xi, 59, 78, 81, 87, 168
laboratory tests, 44, 53
lakes, 157
languages, 122
larynx, 146
Latin America, xv, 11, 12, 13, 14, 15, 19, 68, 131, 132, 141, 148
Latvia, 13
LDCs, 157, 158, 159, 161, 162, 164, 165
LDL, xii, 82, 93, 95, 96, 97
leaching, 108
leadership, 50, 55, 59, 60, 66, 101, 156, 165, 167
learners, 156
learning, 155, 156
learning environment, 156
learning outcomes, 155
Lebanon, 13
legal issues, 89
legislation, xvii, 59, 77, 129, 156, 159, 164, 168
leisure time, 99
leukemia, 7
Liberia, 13, 68, 76
life cycle, 43, 58, 82, 161
life expectancy, 61, 142
lifestyle changes, 10, 96
lipids, 25, 83, 97
lipoproteins, 93
liquids, 93
Lithuania, 13, 15
liver, 10, 25, 83, 93
liver cancer, 25
livestock, 154
living conditions, 15, 26
living environment, 142
long-term debt, 164
low risk, 86
low-density lipoprotein, 93
lung cancer, 107, 109, 132
lung disease, 9
lymphoma, 137

M

Macedonia, 13
magnitude, 3
Maillard reaction, 83
majority, xvi, 25, 63, 78, 81, 109
malaria, 155
Malaysia, 13, 21, 134, 151
malignancy, 6
malignant tumors, ix, 6, 7, 8
malnutrition, 28, 73, 154
market access, 165
marketing, xvi, 24, 28, 29, 57, 58, 59, 60, 63, 68, 80, 85, 86, 121
marriage, 156
Marshall Islands, 13
mass, xi, 7, 29, 86, 97, 168, 173
mass media, 86
materials, 5, 67, 86, 88, 157, 160
Mauritania, 13, 76
Mauritius, 13, 76
measles, 167
meat, 29, 92, 93, 96
media, 60, 62, 69, 85, 168
median, 36
medical care, 43, 51, 110
Medicare, 37
medication, 43, 52, 111
medicine, 44, 49, 53
melanoma, 6

mellitus, 9, 10, 21, 36, 82, 131, 135, 140, 141, 143, 149, 151
mental health, 43, 46, 107, 150, 155
mental illness, 6, 16
messages, 57, 86, 121, 122
meta-analysis, 80, 139, 149
metabolic disorder, 9
metabolic syndrome, 132, 134, 136, 144, 146, 151
metabolism, 9
metastasis, 7
Mexico, 13, 17, 28, 36, 48, 69, 81, 88, 132, 141, 149
Middle East, xv, 11, 12, 13, 14, 15, 18, 19
migrants, 151, 158
migration, 20, 159
modelling, 85
moderate activity, 99
modifiable risk factors
  causal web, ix, 74
  cholesterol, ix, 92, 93, 94, 95, 97, 98, 102
  fats, 92, 93, 96, 138
  physical activity, xii, 96, 98, 99, 139, 147, 173
  sugar intake, 83
Moldova, 13
molecular oxygen, 108
molecules, 93
Mongolia, 13
monounsaturated fatty acids, 93
Montenegro, 13
morbidity, 36, 65, 107, 109, 111, 133, 143, 151
Morocco, xv, 13, 20
mortality, ix, xvii, 24, 28, 30, 32, 36, 55, 61, 65, 78, 80, 95, 107, 109, 110, 111, 113, 117, 120, 123, 125, 131, 133, 139, 141, 142, 143, 154, 155
mortality rate, 131
Mozambique, 14, 76, 99
multi-ethnic, 83, 148
multinational companies, 67
muscles, 10
mutant, 109
mutations, 7
Myanmar, 14, 20, 21, 149
myocardial infarction, 110, 148
myocardium, 110

N

Namibia, 14, 76
narcotic, 155
National Health and Nutrition Examination Survey (NHANES), xii, 82
national income, xii, 15, 16, 21, 45
National Institutes of Health, xii, 37
national policy, 119
national product, 58
national strategy, 81
natural disaster, 62, 161
natural resources, 153, 156, 160
Nauru, 126
negative effects, 69, 168
negotiating, 161
negotiation, 59, 162
neoplasm, 6
Nepal, 14, 20
nerve, 9, 75
nervous system, 7, 93
Netherlands, 14, 91
neutral, 163
New Zealand, xvi, 14, 100, 102
NGOs, xii, xvii, 5, 58, 62, 67, 68, 69, 120, 129, 167
Nicaragua, 14
Nigeria, 14, 36, 37, 47, 75, 76, 117
nitrogen, 109, 150
nitrogen dioxide, 150
North Africa, xv, 11, 12, 13, 14, 15, 18, 19
North America, 11, 15, 18, 123
Norway, 14, 30
nursing, 44
nutrient(s), 59, 83, 84, 91, 132, 162
nutrition, vii, ix, xi, xv, 3, 26, 27, 28, 29, 48, 58, 59, 69, 73, 79, 81, 86, 87, 89, 92, 111, 113, 131, 132, 134, 137, 138, 140, 145, 147, 172, 173
nutrition labels, 69
nutrition transition, 28, 131

O

obesity, 10, 25, 26, 28, 33, 58, 67, 69, 74, 75, 98, 113, 125, 126, 132, 133, 134, 135, 137, 138, 140, 142, 143, 145, 146, 147, 167
obesity prevention, 69
oceans, 162
OECD, xii, 11, 12, 13, 14, 15, 73, 146
Official Development Assistance, xii, 56
olive oil, 74, 96
omega-3, ix, 93, 94, 96
opportunities, 6, 21, 24, 57, 58, 59, 89, 100, 132, 136, 137, 140, 143, 154, 156, 163
oral cavity, 146
organ, 6, 96
organs, 6, 7, 10
osteogenic sarcoma, 134
outpatient, 35, 43, 95, 149
outreach, 43
overproduction, 111
oversight, 41
overweight, 25, 26, 28, 75, 96, 123, 148

ownership, 124, 153, 156
oxidation, 83
oxygen, 92, 108, 110
ozone, xvi, 107, 108, 109, 110, 113, 133, 135, 138, 143, 150
ozone layer, 108

P

pain, xvi, 38
Pakistan, 14, 22, 36, 37, 141
PAL, xii, 100
palliative, 43, 46
Panama, 14
pancreas, 10
Paraguay, 14
pasta, 95
pathogenesis, 144
per capita income, 15, 36
peri-urban, 98, 160
personal relations, 38, 43
personal relationship, 38, 43
persons with disabilities, 156, 158, 160
Peru, 14, 28
pharmaceutical, 5, 63
pharynx, 146
Philippines, 14, 22, 44, 139
phototoxicity, 109
physical activity, xvi, 16, 21, 24, 28, 58, 59, 62, 67, 69, 73, 90, 94, 95, 96, 97, 98, 99, 100, 101, 102, 111, 118, 120, 121, 122, 125, 126, 132, 133, 137, 139, 143, 144, 146, 147, 149, 151, 168, 173, 174
physical education, 168
physical environment, 58
physical inactivity, xv, 6, 10, 21, 24, 25, 26, 28, 29, 60, 66, 73, 98, 102, 118, 120, 135, 139, 142, 167
physical well-being, 24
physicians, 44, 68, 119
phytosterols, 96
planning restrictions, 85
plants, 154
Poland, 14
policy makers, xvii, 110, 129
policy options, 80, 102
policymakers, 99
political system, 24
politics, 42, 63
pollutant, 109
pollutants, 147
pollution, xvii, 25, 68, 107, 109, 111, 113, 132, 133, 142, 150, 151, 157, 162
polycyclic aromatic hydrocarbon, 109
polyunsaturated fatty acids, 93
popular support, 59
population, vii, ix, xv, 17, 20, 21, 22, 23, 24, 28, 29, 30, 32, 41, 44, 46, 48, 49, 60, 61, 75, 78, 80, 81, 88, 95, 99, 102, 111, 113, 117, 118, 122, 123, 125, 129, 131, 132, 134, 139, 151, 159, 168
population growth, ix, 20, 23, 29
population size, vii, 21
Portugal, 14
positive correlation, 82
potassium, 75, 81
potato, 81
poultry, 96
poverty, 26, 56, 60, 153, 163, 165
poverty eradication, 153, 165
poverty reduction, 163
precipitation, 103
pregnancy, 10
premature death, 6, 17, 35, 60, 61, 75
preparedness, 119
preschool, 88, 138
preschool children, 138
prevention, viii, ix, xi, xiii, xvi, xvii, 3, 6, 41, 43, 44, 46, 47, 48, 50, 52, 55, 57, 58, 59, 60, 61, 62, 65, 66, 68, 69, 73, 74, 80, 81, 86, 98, 102, 111, 113, 118, 121, 122, 123, 124, 126, 127, 129, 130, 132, 133, 135, 138, 139, 140, 141, 143, 145, 146, 150, 155, 161, 168, 169
pricing policies, xvii, 129
private sector, 57, 61, 62, 67, 81, 119, 123, 147, 167
probability, 36, 60, 73, 118, 123
procurement, 86, 89, 161
production function, 30
productive capacity, 154
professionals, xvii, 5, 44, 65, 86, 129
programming, 61
prostate cancer, 48, 107
psychosocial stress, 26
public awareness, 86
public education, xvii, 129, 168
public finance, 57
public health, 44, 48, 49, 52, 55, 57, 58, 59, 65, 81, 103, 119, 121, 122, 126, 129, 137, 139, 144, 145, 155
public life, 156
public resources, 48, 56, 119
public schools, 121
public sector, 69
public service, 156
public-private partnerships, 69
Puerto Rico, 14
pulmonary embolism, 6, 109
purchasing power, 59

Q

quality improvement, 141
quality of life, 6, 17, 51, 100
Queensland, 68, 90
questionnaire, 147

R

radiation, 45, 103, 108, 109, 139
radiation therapy, 45
radiation treatment, 45
radiotherapy, 45, 54, 131
rainfall, 108
ratification, 168
reactive oxygen, 83, 146
receptor, 144
recognition, 45
recovery, 163
recreational, 168
recycling, 157, 161
reform(s), 47, 48, 50, 132, 139, 141, 156
regional integration, 167
regions of the world, xvi, 25, 102
regulations, 84, 133, 159
rehabilitation, 43, 46, 47
relief, 164
religion, 159
remittances, 160
renal replacement therapy, 37
renewable energy, 157
renin, 139
Republic of the Congo, 76
requirement9s0, 79, 88, 121
researchers, 5, 21, 33, 80, 88, 89, 98, 110, 123
reserves, 154
resilience, 153, 160, 161, 162
resistance, 59, 60, 83
resource allocation, 50, 134
resources, xvi, xvii, 24, 41, 46, 47, 49, 50, 55, 56, 57, 63, 66, 68, 88, 102, 107, 119, 129, 131, 138, 153, 154, 162, 163, 168
response, 41, 50, 52, 58, 61, 67, 79, 83, 86, 118, 120, 133, 134, 146, 161
restaurants, 78, 79
restoration, 162
restrictions, 85, 154
restructuring, 51, 161, 164
retail, 85, 87, 160
retention rate, 44
reticulum, 140, 146
rheumatic fever, 6
rheumatic heart disease, 6, 109
rings, 66
risk, ix, xv, xvii, 3, 6, 20, 21, 23, 24, 25, 26, 29, 33, 47, 60, 61, 62, 65, 66, 68, 73, 74, 75, 79, 80, 82, 86, 88, 90, 91, 94, 95, 96, 97, 99, 102, 109, 110, 111, 113, 119, 124, 125, 126, 127, 129, 130, 131, 132, 133, 134, 135, 136, 138, 139, 140, 141, 142, 143, 144, 145, 149, 151, 155, 160, 167, 168, 169, 174
risk assessment, 82, 134, 142
risk benefit, 97
risk factors, ix, xv, 3, 6, 20, 21, 23, 24, 25, 26, 29, 60, 61, 62, 73, 74, 86, 90, 102, 111, 119, 124, 126, 130, 131, 136, 138, 140, 142, 167, 168, 169, 174
risk management, 160
Romania, 14
rule of law, 163
rules, 84, 85, 165
rules of origin, 165
runoff, 108
rural areas, 50, 67, 160
Russia, 19, 36, 137
Rwanda, 14, 47, 76

S

safety, 160
Samoa, 14
sanctions, 69
SAR, 13
saturated fat, 29, 73, 74, 91, 93, 94, 95, 96, 102, 111
saturated fatty acids, 74, 93
Saudi Arabia, 14, 35, 131
scaling, 57, 60
scarcity, 113, 157
schistosomiasis, 141
science, 81, 122, 162, 164
scientific knowledge, 162
scientific publications, 5
scope, 3
SEA, 18
sea level, 104
seafood, 96
secondary education, 155
secretion, 10, 83
security, xv, 19, 58, 59, 150
sedentary lifestyle, 24
seed, 154
segregation, 48
self-monitoring, 45
sellers, 92
sensitivity, 9

Serbia, 14
serum, 93, 94, 95, 102, 144
service industries, 24
service organization, 41
service provider, 41
settlements, 160
sex, vii, 76, 159
Seychelles, 14, 76
shellfish, 93
shortage, 45, 50
showing, ix, 105
SIDS, 157, 159, 162, 165
Sierra Leone, 14, 76
Singapore, 14, 20
siphon, 9
skin, 6, 7, 109
skin cancer, 109
SKN, 171, 172, 173, 174, 175
smog, 109
smoking, 6, 21, 73, 97, 168
smoking cessation, 73, 97
social change, 24
social sciences, 5
Social Security, 61
social services, 48
social support, 69
societal cost, 134
society, 28, 69, 148
sodium, vii, ix, 75, 76, 77, 78, 79, 80, 81, 96, 97, 125, 139, 143, 145, 146
soil pollution, 155
Solomon I, 14
Somalia, 14, 30, 76
South Africa, xvi, 14, 19, 33, 41, 46, 49, 50, 75, 76, 79, 81, 98, 101, 102, 123, 134, 138, 140, 141, 142, 143, 144, 145, 147
South America, 21, 132
South Asia, xv, 11, 13, 14, 19, 29, 104
South Korea, 37
Southeast Asia, 21, 131, 143
soymilk, 89
Spain, 14, 61, 62, 124, 134, 167, 171
specialists, 44, 100
species, 83, 146, 154, 163
spending, 30, 35, 36, 45, 46, 56, 57, 61, 149, 159
spinal cord, 7
sputum, 9
squamous cell, 109
Sri Lanka, 14, 21, 45
SSA, 46, 95
stability, 165
stakeholders, xvii, 3, 78, 81, 84, 126, 129
state intervention, 50
state schools, 90
states, 10, 49, 61, 80, 156, 159, 162
statistics, 117, 123, 150
storage, 28, 108
storms, xvii, 104, 111, 113
streptococcal bacteria, 6
stress, xvii, 21, 41, 101, 109, 110, 113, 140
stroke, 22, 25, 33, 74, 75, 76, 78, 94, 97, 102, 107, 109, 110, 123, 137, 138, 139, 167
structure, ix, 3, 6, 51, 93, 94
style, 96, 168
subgroups, 99
sub-Saharan Africa, xvi, 44, 46, 54, 95, 102, 132
substance abuse, 155
substitutes, 88
Sudan, 14, 15, 36, 45, 76, 137
sulphur, 150
supply chain, 86, 160
support services, 51
surveillance, 95, 99, 118, 139, 169, 175
survival, 10
sustainability, 103, 161, 164
sustainable development, xvi, xvii, 3, 54, 55, 57, 129, 140, 153, 156, 161, 162, 163, 164, 165
sustainable energy, 157
Sweden, 15
sweeteners, 29, 82, 83, 89
Switzerland, 15, 46, 131
Syria, 45
systolic blood pressure, 78, 101

T

Taiwan, 15, 36, 135, 151
Tajikistan, 15
talent, 67
Tanzania, 15, 76, 98, 138
target, 43, 61, 79, 80, 126, 148
target population, 43
Task Force, xiii, 58, 60, 61
tax collection, 57
taxation, 161
taxes, 56, 57, 59, 69, 84, 85, 88, 138, 172
teacher training, 156
teachers, 156
technical assistance, 55, 89, 160
technical support, 159
techniques, 28, 85
technological advances, 24, 28, 29
technological change, 24
technology, 48, 122, 153, 154, 156, 157, 159, 162, 164
temperature, 103, 104, 107, 108, 109, 143, 146

terrorism, 164
tertiary education, 155
Thailand, 15, 21, 36, 81, 135, 139, 140, 145, 146
therapy, 137
threats, 103
thrombosis, 6, 109
time periods, 103, 104
tissue, 7
tobacco, xv, xvii, 24, 25, 29, 56, 57, 59, 60, 61, 62, 122, 125, 126, 129, 141, 142, 167, 168
Togo, 15, 76
Tonga, 15
torture, 163
total cholesterol, 95, 96, 97
total costs, 35
total energy, 73, 82, 83, 100
tourism, 158, 161, 162
trade, 24, 57, 60, 87, 111, 154, 168
trafficking, 156, 163
training, 44, 45, 49, 53, 67, 68, 79, 119, 127, 155, 158
transaction costs, 160
translation, 52, 149
transparency, 161
transplantation, 37
transport, 49, 99, 111, 113, 146, 150, 160
transportation, 111
Treasury, 61
treatment, xvii, 6, 33, 35, 41, 43, 44, 45, 47, 48, 54, 55, 58, 61, 119, 120, 124, 126, 147, 155, 157, 174
triglycerides, 83
Trinidad, xv, 15, 20, 62, 123, 124, 134, 167, 175
Trinidad and Tobago, xv, 15, 20, 62, 123, 134, 167, 175
tuberculosis, 50, 155
tumor, 6, 7
Turkey, 15
Turkmenistan, 15
Turks, 15, 175
Tuvalu, 15
type 2 diabetes, vii, 36, 73, 80, 82, 98, 111, 113, 135, 138, 140, 141, 143, 144, 145, 146, 149

U

U.S. economy, 33
Ukraine, 15
UNFCCC, 161
uninsured, 48
United Kingdom, 15, 37, 78, 111, 147
United Nations, xiii, 20, 22, 23, 60, 61, 103, 125, 138, 145, 148
universal access, 49, 50, 155, 156, 157, 160
urban areas, 20, 21, 44, 103, 117, 118
urban population, 28, 150
urban settlement, 151
urbanicity, 21, 136, 149
urbanization, xv, 21, 23, 24, 28, 29, 60, 68, 82, 111, 131, 139, 143, 151, 160
uric acid, 144
urine, 45
Uruguay, 15, 37
UV radiation, 108, 109
Uzbekistan, 15

V

validation, 147
Vanuatu, 15
variations, 103
vector, 110
vegetable oil, 29, 96
vegetables, 26, 28, 73, 83, 84, 91, 92, 95, 96, 97, 122, 126
vehicles, 168
vein, 6, 109
Venezuela, 15, 35, 126
vessels, 6
Vietnam, 15, 21, 45, 133, 140
violence, 156, 163, 164
vision, 6, 41
vitamin D, 93
vitamins, 83
VLDL, 93
vocational training, 156
volatile organic compounds, 109
volatility, 154
volatilization, 108
vulnerability, 111, 135, 139, 140, 147, 153

W

wages, 44
walking, 67, 99
waste management, 160
wastewater, 157
water, 45, 48, 89, 90, 92, 103, 107, 108, 113, 155, 157, 160, 161, 163
water ecosystems, 163
water quality, 45, 157
water resources, 157
water vapor, 103
wavelengths, 108
weather patterns, 103
web, ix, 5, 73, 74

web pages, 5
weight control, 94, 102
weight gain, 73, 91, 146
weight loss, 10, 96
weight status, 147
well-being, 100, 155, 158, 167
wellness, 143, 168
West Bank, 15
West Indies, 149
wetlands, 157, 162
wheezing, 9
workers, ix, xvii, 33, 34, 44, 47, 49, 53, 57, 67, 119, 121, 126, 127, 129, 158, 159
workforce, 24, 33, 44, 53, 67, 155
World Bank, vii, xv, 5, 11, 15, 16, 19, 46, 56, 58, 76, 104, 117, 134, 144, 151
World Development Report, 104
World Health Organization (WHO), xiii, xv, xvi, 5, 6, 9, 17, 19, 20, 21, 25, 26, 28, 41, 43, 45, 46, 47, 49, 50, 51, 52, 55, 56, 57, 58, 59, 60, 61, 63, 73, 75, 79, 80, 81, 82, 83, 94, 95, 98, 99, 102, 103, 106, 109, 113, 117, 118, 119, 121, 122, 123, 125, 126, 132, 134, 139, 141, 144, 146, 150, 167
worldwide, x, 24, 29, 50, 107, 109, 132, 142, 145
WTO, xiii, 57, 159, 162, 165

Y

Yemen, 15
yolk, 93
young people, 98, 99, 100, 158

Z

Zimbabwe, 15, 76